T0144660

BASIC HEALTH PUBLICATIONS USER'S GUIDE

TO PREVENTING & REVERSING DIABETES NATURALLY

Learn How to Use
Foods & Supplements
to Protect Against
Blood-Sugar
Disorders.

MELISSA DIANE SMITH

JACK CHALLEM Series Editor

The information contained in this book is based upon the research and personal and professional experiences of the author. It is not intended as a substitute for consulting with your physician or other healthcare provider. Any attempt to diagnose and treat an illness should be done under the direction of a healthcare professional.

The publisher does not advocate the use of any particular healthcare protocol but believes the information in this book should be available to the public. The publisher and author are not responsible for any adverse effects or consequences resulting from the use of the suggestions, preparations, or procedures discussed in this book. Should the reader have any questions concerning the appropriateness of any procedures or preparations mentioned, the author and the publisher strongly suggest consulting a professional healthcare advisor.

Series Editor: Jack Challem
Editor: Tara Durkin
Typesetter: Gary A. Rosenberg
Series Cover Designer: Mike Stromberg

Basic Health Publications User's Guides are published by Basic Health Publications, Inc.

ISBN: 978-1-59120-094-9 (Pbk.)
ISBN: 978-1-68162-867-7 (Hardcover)

CONTENTS

*For my Greek grandfather
who had "a little bit of sugar"
at the end of his life*

INTRODUCTION

Most of us are concerned about heart disease and cancer, the two leading causes of death in our society, and we give little thought to diabetes. But we should. Diabetes is the fastest-growing deadly disease, and it increases the risk of these other major killers.

In diabetes (specifically type 2 diabetes), the body is not able to properly use the food we eat to supply energy to our cells. It was long thought to develop only in older adults, but the incidence of diabetes has skyrocketed in all age groups in the past decade or so. Today, children as young as ten years old are developing this silent killer, and the biggest jump in numbers has occurred in people in their thirties.

What's more, diabetes usually takes years to develop. Millions of people already have some type of prediabetes, such as Syndrome X, which includes abdominal obesity, high blood pressure, and unhealthy cholesterol and triglyceride levels. Millions more—almost two-thirds of the United States population—are overweight, which is *the* major risk factor for developing diabetes. It's apparent that all of us should be thinking about what we can do to prevent diabetes and all the serious complications that accompany it—or how we can control or reverse the condition if we've already been diagnosed with it.

And there's plenty we can do. The twin epidemics of diabetes and excess weight have become public health problems because of a combination of poor diet, excessive stress, and lack of physical activity—all factors that are well within our ability to control and change. At the top of the list is diet. Diabetes and prediabetes are first and foremost nutritional diseases: they respond amazingly well to a lower-carbohydrate diet and thoughtful use of nutritional supplements.

It turns out that the key to controlling the serious complications that usually occur with diabetes—maintaining healthy blood sugar levels—is also the key to promoting good health and a long life. So, whether you have diabetes, are at risk for developing it, or simply want to know the latest on how to maintain or improve your health, sit back, read through this guide, and give yourself a healthy edge.

CHAPTER 1

WHY *EVERYONE* SHOULD BE CONCERNED ABOUT DIABETES

Diabetes and the disease process that leads to it are so common—and the consequences so serious—that all of us should be concerned about protecting ourselves against it. Diabetes is the sixth leading cause of death in the United States (by some estimates, the third leading cause), and its prevalence continues to increase at alarming rates in both sexes, all ages, all races, and all education levels.

An estimated 16 to 17 million Americans have diabetes, and perhaps one-third to one-half of these people don't know it. Millions more have some type of prediabetes, usually without knowing it, including many of the 65 percent of Americans who are overweight.

The increased prevalence of diabetes has paralleled the steady expansion of Americans' waistlines over the past decade. However, even if you are of normal weight and have no special risk for diabetes, you should know that the standard American diet (appropriately abbreviated SAD) sets us up for excess weight, diabetes, and prediabetes, if not in the short term then in the long term. It's important to take steps now to avoid becoming one of these statistics.

The Most Common and Fastest-Growing Type of Diabetes

There are two main types of diabetes. This book is

all about type 2 diabetes, the most common and the fastest-growing type. Type 2 affects 90 to 95 percent of people who have been diagnosed with diabetes and most of the millions more who are at risk for developing it.

Insulin is the hormone the body produces to lower blood sugar levels (and move sugar into cells where it becomes energy). In type 1 diabetes, the pancreas stops producing adequate insulin because of a malfunction in the immune system. Insulin shots, therefore, are needed for the rest of the person's life.

Type 2 Diabetes
The most common and fastest-growing type of diabetes. Develops from blood-sugar-lowering insulin's not working properly.

Type 2 diabetes starts out very differently. Usually, the body makes plenty of insulin but doesn't use it properly: the cells aren't receptive to insulin's blood-sugar-lowering actions. (In later, more advanced stages of type 2 diabetes, though, the pancreas eventually tires of pumping out so much insulin and stops producing adequate amounts.)

Type 2 diabetes was long called adult-onset diabetes because the condition was usually only diagnosed in people who were middle-aged or older. But that term is now passé because type 2 diabetes is quickly becoming a disease of the young as well as the old. A more detailed explanation of how diabetes and prediabetes develop follows in Chapter 2, but it's best to think of type 2 diabetes as "insulin-resistant diabetes."

Are You at Risk?

Type 2 diabetes is often called "the silent killer" because it develops gradually and can cause serious health complications. However, many people do not even know they have diabetes or that they are at risk for developing it. Research shows that by the time a person is diagnosed with type 2 diabetes, he or she has probably been developing the condition for at least eight to twelve years. Furthermore, in 50 percent of cases the patient has serious health complications by the time of diagnosis.

It's important to know if you're one of the growing number of people who is at risk of developing diabetes. Read over the following risk factors and check all that apply:

❏ I am 10–15 pounds or more overweight.

❏ I have high blood pressure.

❏ I have increased blood triglycerides.

❏ I have low high-density lipoprotein (HDL) cholesterol.

❏ I have cardiovascular disease.

❏ I have slightly high blood sugar levels or have tested positive for impaired glucose tolerance.

❏ I lead an inactive lifestyle.

❏ I am an African American, Hispanic, Pacific Islander, or Native American.

❏ I have a family history of diabetes.

For women only:

❏ I have, or have had, gestational diabetes (a temporary type of diabetes that develops during pregnancy).

❏ I have given birth to a baby weighing more than 9 pounds.

❏ I have polycystic ovary syndrome (or PCOS, which is characterized by symptoms such as irregular menstrual periods, difficulty getting pregnant, and excessive facial hair).

Polycystic Ovary Syndrome *An insulin-related condition that affects females, causing ovarian cysts, irregular menstrual periods, excess facial hair, and sometimes infertility.*

If you checked even one of the factors above, you are at increased risk of developing diabetes. Based on evidence showing that the greatest jump in the incidence of diabetes has recently occurred among people in their thirties, the American College of Endocrinology now recommends that anyone with any risk factor above be screened for the disease by age thirty. The more risk factors you have, of course, the more important it is that you're checked—not just once, but regularly—for diabetes.

A Diet with Refined Carbohydrates— The Biggest Risk Factor

There's one more risk factor for diabetes and it's a big one: eating a diet high in refined carbohydrates—that is, white flour (found in bread, pasta, and baked goods), white rice, white sugar, and other sweeteners (such as high-fructose corn syrup and most food ingredients ending in –ose). Consider that one 1997 study found that women who eat large amounts of refined carbohydrates have double the risk of developing diabetes, compared with those who eat fewer refined foods. What's more, a high intake of refined carbohydrates also can lead to the development of virtually all of the health conditions that are diabetes risk factors, including packing on the pounds and becoming overweight. (You'll learn more about this process in Chapter 2.)

Even if you have an increased risk of diabetes, understand that diabetes is first and foremost a nutritional disease. Don't convince yourself that there's nothing you can do to prevent the disease or that genetics are destiny. Here are the facts: In the past several decades, when the prevalence of excess weight and diabetes has increased by unheard-of numbers, our genes haven't changed. But our diet has—and dramatically. Our intake of dietary fat actually has decreased, but our intake of grains (mainly refined grains) has increased by more than 60 pounds per person per year, and our intake of sugar has increased by 30 pounds per person per year. Our intake of grains and sugars is the single biggest change to account for the record numbers of people who are overweight and who have diabetes. Given that diabetes is characterized by high blood sugar levels, it only makes sense that a diet high in refined carbohydrates, which break down into sugars quickly, greatly increases the risk of developing the disease.

The Fattening of the World and the Spread of Diabetes

Because our refined-carbohydrate foods have spread to other lands, people around the world have gradually developed the same health problems with obesity and diabetes that we have. Worldwide, 300 million people are obese and 750 million are overweight, according to World Health Organization (WHO) officials. Especially troubling is that in some areas of the developing world, more children are afflicted by fatness and obesity than malnutrition.

Fatness and obesity are not simply cosmetic problems: they cut years off people's lives. Being fat at forty reduces life expectancy by at least three years—as much as smoking cigarettes. Obese people lose even more years, about six or seven according to recent studies. The younger people are when they pack on the pounds, the more years they stand to lose, up to as many as twenty.

Being overweight increases the risk of numerous chronic diseases, including cardiovascular disease, high blood pressure, high cholesterol levels, asthma, arthritis, and cancer. But it is diabetes that health experts are most concerned about.

Fatness and diabetes tend to go had in hand: 85 percent of all people with diabetes are overweight or obese, and the fatter people become, the greater their risk of developing diabetes. There's a delay between the development of obesity and the onset of diabetes, which means that for many overweight and obese people it is just a matter of time before the disease sets in.

About 177 million people worldwide have diabetes today, but that figure is expected to surpass 300 million by 2025. Experts such as Dr. Paul Zimmet, director of the International Diabetes Institute in Victoria, Australia, predict that diabetes is going to be the biggest epidemic in human history.

Complications of Diabetes

Diabetes is an epidemic that comes with a high price. The long-term complications that can develop are many and serious, including the following:

Amputations

Diabetes is the second most frequent cause of lower-limb amputations after accidental injuries. The risk of a leg amputation is fifteen to forty times greater for a person with diabetes.

Blindness (Retinopathy)

Diabetes is the leading cause of new cases of blindness among adults between the ages of twenty and seventy-four. Up to 24,000 Americans will go blind this year due to complications from diabetes.

Complications of Pregnancy

Poorly controlled diabetes before conception and during the first trimester of pregnancy can cause major birth defects in 5 to 10 percent of pregnancies and miscarriages in 15 to 20 percent of pregnancies. Poorly controlled diabetes during the second and third trimesters can result in excessively large babies, posing a risk to the mother and child.

Dental Disease

Periodontal or gum diseases are more common among people with diabetes than among people without diabetes. Almost one-third of people with diabetes have severe periodontal diseases with loss of gum-to-teeth attachment measuring 5 millimeters or more.

Heart Disease and Stroke

People with diabetes are two to four times more likely to have heart disease and to suffer a stroke. More significantly, heart disease is the leading cause of diabetes-related deaths: *Eight out of ten people with diabetes die from a cardiovascular disease.*

Kidney Damage (Nephropathy)

Diabetes is the leading cause of end-stage kidney disease, accounting for 43 percent of new cases. This complication often requires a kidney transplant or dialysis (which are both stressful, complicated, and expensive treatments) for survival.

Nerve Damage (Neuropathy)

Sixty to 70 percent of people with diabetes suffer mild to severe nerve damage that causes a tingling, burning, or numbing sensation in the feet and/or hands, carpal tunnel syndrome (in the hand

and wrist), digestive ailments, or sexual problems (such as erectile dysfunction in men or difficulty in reaching full sexual climax in both men and women). Severe forms of diabetic nerve disease are a major contributing cause of lower-extremity amputations.

Other Illnesses

People with diabetes have an increased risk of developing several types of cancer, such as colorectal, prostate, breast, and endometrial cancers. They also are more susceptible to various other illnesses, and, once they acquire these illnesses, their prognosis is worse than if they did not have diabetes. For example, people with diabetes are more likely to die from pneumonia or influenza than people without diabetes who develop these illnesses.

Perhaps most importantly, the risk of death among people with diabetes is about two times greater than that of people without diabetes.

Furthermore, these serious complications aren't just seen in adults. The first group of children diagnosed with type 2 diabetes has grown up, and their experiences clearly show how serious this disease is. A study that tracked the fifty-one former children (who are now between eighteen and thirty-three years old) reported one toe amputation, one case of blindness, and a high rate of miscarriage (38 percent), dialysis (6 percent), and death (9 percent).

The High Price of Diabetes

The costs of the disease are exceptionally high—not just in personal terms, but in monetary terms as well. Tallying up direct medical expenses and indirect expenses (including work loss, disability, and premature death), the cost of diabetes in the United States is estimated to be almost $100 billion. That figure is expected only to get worse. If obesity and diabetes trends continue at their current rates, the impact on our nation's and our world's business and healthcare costs in the future will be overwhelming, if not crippling. Fortunately, those trends can be reversed.

Diabetes Is Preventable and Controllable

There is good news in all of this: A good nutritional and lifestyle program not only can prevent diabetes but also can control it and, in most cases, reverse it if you already have the condition. Maintaining healthy blood sugar levels is the key to preventing the serious health complications that usually come with diabetes and to promoting good health in general. It is easy to maintain normal blood sugar by following the suggestions offered in this book.

How effective is good blood sugar control for people who have diabetes? Very. Just in terms of work alone, people with diabetes who improve their blood sugar control take fewer sick days, are more productive on the job, have fewer days of restricted activity, and are able to remain employed longer than employees who do not control and lower their blood sugar levels. This translates into more income for the employee and greater work efficiency for the employer.

In terms of health, good blood sugar control can reverse many cases of diabetes, helping diabetic patients reduce or eliminate medications. Moreover, it can promote long-term good health and prevent the disease from developing in the first place. Even in long-term cases of diabetes, the condition can be controlled and all of the life-threatening complications can be held at bay.

The next chapter will give you more details

about blood sugar function, so that you will know what to watch out for and can be more prepared to protect yourself against diabetes and pre-diabetes.

CHAPTER 2

BASICS ABOUT DIABETES AND PREDIABETES

Diabetes doesn't develop overnight. Minor problems in blood sugar function start slowly and imperceptibly, gradually leading to bigger problems and eventually to prediabetes and diabetes.

As already mentioned, the standard American diet, high in refined carbohydrates, sets us up for blood sugar imbalance. Consequently, many people today have blood sugar problems of one type or another and are at risk of developing diabetes, even though they don't know it. This chapter will help you understand one of the most important self-regulating systems of the body—blood sugar function—and how to catch early signs of blood sugar imbalance, prediabetes, and diabetes.

Blood Sugar 101

Every time we eat carbohydrates—which are found in foods such as grains, sugars, beans, vegetables, and fruits—our body breaks them down into glucose, a type of sugar that serves as the body's main fuel. Our body functions best when blood sugar (or blood glucose) levels stay steady in normal ranges, so the body works hard to maintain a fairly even stream of glucose in the blood.

Since blood sugar levels rise after eating, a common test of blood sugar function is a fasting blood glucose test, taken in the morning before eating. A normal fasting blood glucose is between

65 and 110 mg/dl (milligrams per deciliter), but an optimal range is considered by many blood-sugar-savvy health professionals to be between 75 and 90 mg/dl. When fasting blood sugar levels are consistently high, this is an indicator of diabetes, and moderately high fasting blood sugar levels often help determine prediabetes.

After you eat, blood sugar levels initially rise and then decline slowly. This is referred to by doctors as your "postprandial" (or postmeal) curve. Normally, this curve should be between 65 and 139 mg/dl. Very high postmeal blood sugar levels (in addition to high fasting blood sugar levels) are another common indicator of diabetes. Moderately high curves can signal prediabetes. A very modest increase in your postmeal blood sugar curve is normal: this indicates good blood sugar function.

Insulin Governs Blood Sugar Levels

So, what determines how much glucose stays in your blood? A number of hormones are involved, but insulin is the key one.

Insulin
A key metabolic hormone that lowers blood sugar levels by increasing the rate that glucose is taken up by cells throughout the body.

When we eat carbohydrates, our body responds by signaling the pancreas, a gland located in the back of the abdominal cavity, to secrete insulin. Insulin works like a key, opening the cell door and allowing glucose to enter so that glucose can be burned in energy-producing reactions within our cells. If insulin isn't working efficiently, glucose is not removed from the bloodstream (glucose does not get into the cells), blood sugar levels rise, and diabetes results.

Diet Can Make or Break Blood Sugar Function

Blood sugar function usually works very smoothly

when we eat foods that release glucose slowly into the bloodstream—think fish or poultry and lots of steamed broccoli and salad. These are modern-day versions of the types of whole foods our distant ancestors ate. But blood sugar function goes awry when we consistently eat foods that cause high spikes in blood sugar levels. Unfortunately, that's what North Americans (and more and more people around the world) have been doing for quite some time.

Refined-grain-based foods, such as bread, muffins, crackers, and cookies, became a part of the typical American diet only about a century ago, and as the years went on, they became an increasingly larger part. The problem is that refined grains act just like sugar in the body, prompting sharp rises in blood sugar levels. (Our intake of sugar, which obviously prompts sharp rises in blood sugar levels, has skyrocketed as well.) So, the more we've eaten refined grains and sugars, the more we've run into health problems associated with imbalanced blood sugar function, especially diabetes.

The Diabetes Disease Process

Specifically, what happens in the body is this: High-carbohydrate foods, such as sweets, breads, and flour- and sugar-based snack foods, trigger a rapid increase in blood sugar levels. High levels of blood sugar are toxic to the kidneys and other organs, so the pancreas responds by pumping out high amounts of blood-sugar-regulating insulin to deal with all the extra blood sugar. Insulin converts a portion of the excess glucose into glycogen, a storage form of sugar in the muscles and liver. Once glycogen storage areas are filled and there is still more glucose in the blood beyond that which the body needs to function, insulin will convert the excess to fat. That's why the large amount of carbohydrates in the typical American diet is leading to millions of people becoming overweight. Insulin is a premier fat-storage hormone.

Over time, the body's cells become overwhelmed by so much insulin and actually become resistant (or not very receptive) to it. This condition, known as insulin resistance, forces the pancreas to work harder to produce enough insulin to maintain blood sugar at close to normal ranges. (Think of the analogy of taking so much of a drug that the drug loses its effectiveness and you have to take more of it to get the same effect.)

Insulin Resistance
A condition in which the body does not respond to insulin efficiently. High insulin levels typically accompany insulin resistance.

The combination of insulin resistance and high insulin levels can go on for years without a person realizing it because blood sugar levels may be normal or near normal. But the excess insulin the pancreas is continually pumping out starts doing damage to the body, altering blood-fat ratios, raising blood pressure, and increasing fat storage, especially through the middle of the body.

Syndrome X
Insulin resistance plus abdominal obesity, high blood pressure, high blood triglycerides, and/or unhealthy blood cholesterol levels.

This can lead to a more advanced form of insulin resistance in which abdominal obesity, high blood pressure, high triglycerides, and/or unhealthy cholesterol levels (low HDL or poor LDL-to-HDL ratios) are also present. This cluster of heart-disease risk factors is a condition known as Syndrome X, or the insulin-resistance syndrome. Each of the components of Syndrome X increases the risk of not just heart disease but diabetes as well. The more of these heart-disease risk factors you have, the more at risk you are.

Some people go on to develop diabetes and some don't. In those who don't, their bodies keep pumping out high levels of insulin and they could develop heart disease or a number of other diseases associated with high insulin levels, including Alzheimer's disease or pancreatic, liver, breast, or colorectal cancer.

For those who follow the road to diabetes, the normal chain of events is this: As insulin resistance increases, the pancreas loses its ability to respond adequately to meals that are eaten. Therefore, postmeal glucose levels start to rise higher than normal, a condition known as impaired glucose tolerance. Further insulin resistance (which is starving cells of fuel) forces the liver to respond by increasing glucose production, which makes fasting blood glucose levels rise.

Both conditions—fasting or postmeal blood glucose levels that are higher than normal but not high enough to be classified as diabetes—are considered forms of prediabetes. Diabetes is typically diagnosed when glucose levels go even higher.

Prediabetes
Conditions that develop before diabetes, such as Syndrome X and slightly elevated fasting or postmeal blood glucose levels.

Most people with diabetes (meaning type 2 diabetes) produce plenty of insulin, often two to three times the amount that people without diabetes produce. (The insulin, as you'll recall, just isn't working efficiently.) In the later stages of this disease, though, the pancreas becomes so exhausted that it stops producing adequate amounts.

Diagnosing Diabetes and Prediabetes

Much debate is occurring in medical circles about precisely when to diagnose prediabetes and diabetes. The standard criteria are:

Prediabetes: Fasting blood glucose levels between 110 and 125 mg/dl, and two-hour postmeal blood glucose levels (taken two hours after eating) between 140 and 199 mg/dl.

Diabetes: Fasting blood glucose levels above 125 mg/dl, and postmeal glucose levels (taken two hours after eating) above 200 mg/dl.

However, by the time a person has met the postmeal blood glucose criteria for prediabetes, his or her risk of cardiovascular disease is greatly increased. And by the time a person has met the criteria for diabetes, he or she often has already developed serious health complications. Therefore, it is important to catch the diabetes disease process much earlier, before so much damage has taken place in the body.

To help with earlier diagnosis, many doctors use other helpful tests, such as fasting and post-meal blood insulin tests, a fasting C-peptide test (which gives an index of the amount of insulin the body is producing), oral glucose-tolerance tests (in which blood sugar levels are monitored after you drink a sugary solution) and hemoglobin A1c tests (which give an estimate of average blood sugar levels for the past three or four months). These tools can help doctors determine the extent to which blood sugar and insulin function may be impaired.

Watching Out for Signs of Diabetes and Prediabetes

The best way to protect yourself from diabetes and prediabetes is to watch out for warning signs and symptoms and monitor how you feel. Now that you understand the diabetes disease process, you can see that millions of people—including those who have excess weight around the middle (such as a potbelly), those who have high blood pressure, those who have unhealthy cholesterol or triglyceride levels, or those who have slightly elevated blood sugar levels—already have some type of prediabetes. You could be one of them. If you aren't one of these people, that's good. But, still, be on the lookout for other signs of blood sugar imbalance:

- Excessive fatigue

- Tiredness or sleepiness after meals

- Difficulty concentrating

- Frequent cravings for sweets, breads, and other high-carbohydrate foods

- Feeling "high" after eating sugary sweets, followed by feeling low a while later

- Being overweight or having difficulty losing weight

- Irritability if you go too long without eating

Diabetes, of course, is much more serious. If you experience any of the following symptoms, consult your doctor immediately and ask to be tested for the condition:

- Frequent urination

- Excessive thirst

- Extreme hunger

- Blurred vision or any change in eyesight

- Cuts that heal slowly, especially on the hands and feet

- Frequent yeast infections (in women)

- Sudden unexplained weight loss or weight gain

- Tingling sensation or numbness in the legs, feet, or fingers

The Damaging Effects of High Insulin

No matter what blood-sugar-related symptoms and conditions you may have, it's important to understand that high insulin levels and high blood sugar levels wreak havoc in the body, putting you on the fast track to degenerative disease and accelerated aging. Chronically high insulin levels develop earlier in the diabetes disease process than chronically high blood sugar levels, so we'll consider the trouble with high insulin first.

Insulin is a powerful mitogen—that is, it stimulates the division of cells and the activation of genes. Prolonged exposure to high levels of insulin actually accelerates the aging of cells, or makes younger cells act like older cells. It shouldn't be surprising, therefore, that high insulin levels contribute to the development of many of the diseases of aging. As already mentioned, high insulin levels are associated with numerous age-related, chronic conditions—not just diabetes and heart disease, but also cognitive disorders, impaired thinking processes, dementia, Alzheimer's disease, and liver, pancreatic, endometrial, breast, and colorectal cancer.

The Damaging Effects of High Blood Sugar

High blood sugar (or high glucose) also does damage in the body. First, high blood sugar generates large numbers of free radicals—destructive molecules that damage cells and age them. As one example, oxidized low-density cholesterol forms when free radicals attack LDL cholesterol. Oxidized LDL is a much more harmful cholesterol than regular LDL cholesterol: it is so

Free Radicals
Highly unstable molecules that damage and age cells. Produced by the body in higher amounts in people with diabetes and prediabetes.

sticky that it attaches to rough spots on the walls of your arteries and can lead to the formation of plaque and clogged arteries.

Free-radical damage has been linked to virtually all diseases of aging. The more free radicals in the body, without the balance of antioxidants (protective molecules that quench free radicals), the faster cells become damaged, the body ages, and disease sets in.

Excess glucose (or its metabolite, sorbitol) also causes problems in the body because it binds to, chemically alters and damages proteins in organs and tissues. These substances, called "advanced glycation end-products," interfere with normal functioning because they affect the production of thousands of different proteins that your body makes to regulate its functions. The abbreviation for advanced glycation end products, AGEs, is appropriate: AGEs toughen proteins and quite literally age cells.

Glucose that combines with the protein hemoglobin in your blood is glycosylated hemoglobin or hemoglobin A1c, which is what diabetic patients regularly test to monitor control of their condition. Since the average red cell survives about four months, the percentage of hemoglobin molecules that contain glucose can provide an estimate of average blood sugar over this time frame.

Hemoglobin A1c
Sugar-damaged hemoglobin that people with diabetes measure in their blood and use as a marker to monitor control of their condition.

AGEs are involved in diabetic complications of the kidneys and circulatory system, in clouding the proteins in the lens of the eye (forming cataracts), in the formation of plaques found in the brains of those with Alzheimer's disease, and in the development of wrinkled skin and stiff joints. Often it's a combination of AGEs and lots of free radicals that leads to the development of the serious health complications of diabetes.

The damaging effects of even moderately elevated blood sugar also include impaired functioning of white blood cells and lowered resistance to infection over time. If your blood sugar is poorly controlled, you can be more prone to developing serious infections caused by bacteria and fungi that other people aren't bothered by (such as *Candida* yeast infections). Even worse, you can be at increased risk of developing dangerous infections from open wounds that would not pose problems in people with normal blood sugars.

With blood sugar, you don't just run into trouble if your fasting or postmeal blood sugar levels are high enough to qualify as diabetes. "A little bit of sugar"—as people often say when referring to slightly high blood sugar levels—still causes plenty of problems. Prediabetic fasting blood sugar levels (above 110 mg/dl but below 125 mg/dl) greatly increase the risk of diabetes and heart disease. In addition, fasting blood sugar levels in the upper range of normal (say, 109 mg/dl) increase the risk of death from heart disease substantially more than levels at the lower range of normal (say, 80 mg/dl). Recent research out of the Center for Brain Health at the New York University School of Medicine also shows an association between impaired glucose tolerance (prediabetes) and memory problems. Therefore, the more you can lower blood sugar readings toward optimal levels, the least likely you are to age prematurely, to get a fuzzy memory with age, and to die from a heart attack.

The Best Strategy for Health: Controlling Blood Sugar and Insulin

Diabetes and prediabetes are dangerous diseases that should be taken very seriously. For a long time, people with diabetes thought the most life-threatening complications they needed to protect themselves against were high-blood-sugar-induced comas (from uncontrolled, extremely high blood sugar levels) or low-blood-sugar-induced comas (usually brought on from overmedicating with hypoglycemic drugs). We now know that people with diabetes are more likely to die from a long-term complication—brought on by years of high blood sugar and high insulin—than they are to die from a short, crisis-type, acute complication. And we also know that sugar and insulin levels that are only slightly higher than normal can cause silent damage to your system, gradually and cumulatively ruining your health, whether you have diabetes or not.

The lesson? Adopt a lifestyle that keeps blood sugar and insulin levels in healthy ranges, and you'll prevent or reverse the diabetes disease process and keep the body functioning in tip-top shape for years to come.

The rest of the book will help you learn exactly how to do that, starting with the next chapter, which addresses the tremendous importance of diet.

CHAPTER 3

USING FOOD AS MEDICINE: THE IMPORTANCE OF DIET

We've all heard that a good diet is crucial for protecting against diabetes and excess weight—and that food is our best medicine. Unfortunately, few of us really know how to put that strategy into practice.

The secret, as you learned in the last chapter, is to eat in a way that keeps blood sugar and insulin levels in healthy ranges throughout each and every day. This isn't as difficult as it sounds. Just rethink what you may have been taught to believe about food, open your mind to new ideas, and follow the eating guidelines in this chapter. You'll find that blood-sugar-balancing meals are tasty, easy to fix, *and* health promoting.

Cut Carbs: Avoid Sugars, Grains, and Potatoes

With low-carb diets and books in the news, most of us have heard, at least in passing, about the value of reducing carbohydrates for losing weight and controlling diabetes. Carbohydrates are long chains of sugars, so it only makes sense to substantially reduce dietary carbohydrates to control blood sugar and insulin levels. However, some of us have probably gotten the wrong message about the best way to control our carbohydrate intake. The idea isn't to load up on low-carbohydrate processed food all day long, or to use a certain allotment of carbohydrates for the day on anything you want—a sweet, some bread, pasta, or a breakfast bar—and then eat few other carbohydrates the rest of the day. The way to maintain steady blood sugar and insulin levels throughout the day is to eat a little bit of fiber- and nutrient-rich carbohydrates at every meal and to avoid nutrient-poor, blood-sugar-spiking sources of carbohydrates.

As you've already learned, foods made with refined sugars and grains are the worst for blood sugar levels. They are the most important foods to avoid for better health, weight control, and protection against diabetes.

Some health professionals recommend whole-grain foods in place of refined grains, but this is a mistake. Grains, whether whole grain or not, are high in carbohydrates and calories, and they raise blood sugar levels more than most vegetables. They're also used to fatten up cattle and they can do exactly the same to us.

If you're reading this book, the chances are that you're overweight or at risk of developing diabetes. Losing excess fat, or maintaining a healthy weight, is crucial to reducing your risk of diabetes. Avoiding high-carbohydrate foods that can pack on the pounds—sugars, grain products (breads, pasta, and baked goods), and starchy vegetables such as potatoes—is the most foolproof way to lose weight and to keep blood sugar and insulin at healthy levels.

Eat Your Veggies

Grandma knew what she was talking about when she said to eat your veggies. The types of carbohydrates that promote the most minimal rise in blood sugar and insulin levels are nonstarchy vegetables (those that aren't root vegetables or winter squash), such as asparagus, broccoli, cabbage, celery, green beans, peppers, and leafy greens.

They're rich in fiber, which slows release of glucose into the blood, and they're also rich in vitamins and minerals, which the body needs to promote optimal functioning.

A golden rule in nutrition is to get as much nutritional value per calorie that you can. Nonstarchy vegetables are at the top of the carbohydrate list in this regard. On a per-cup or per-serving basis, they have four to forty times fewer carbohydrates than grain-based foods such as pasta. That means you can eat a lot more of nonstarchy vegetables without throwing your blood sugar and insulin levels into unhealthy ranges. One study conducted in Great Britain in 1999 found that men and women who frequently ate salad and raw vegetables year-round had an 80 percent lower risk of diabetes than people who ate vegetables less often.

Get Plenty of Protein

Eating regular amounts of protein—such as chicken, turkey, fish, lean red meats and eggs—is important to balance out the diet and keep you from eating too many carbohydrates. Protein boosts metabolism, helps build and repair muscles, and stimulates the production of glucagon, an insulin-opposing hormone that helps the body burn stored fat. With inadequate protein, your metabolism slows and you lose muscle mass. With adequate protein, you can lose fat and maintain (or build) muscle, which is the only health-promoting way to lose weight.

Blood-sugar-balancing meals of lean animal protein and nonstarchy vegetables or fruit also reduce hunger and overeating; they're the best antidote to an overzealous appetite and carbohydrate cravings. Make this combination of foods a regular feature of all meals, but especially breakfast. When you start your day with an egg and veggie omelet instead of cereal, you will eat fewer calories, feel better, and be far less likely to have a snack attack in between meals.

Contrary to what many people with diabetes have heard, protein does not hurt healthy kidneys or cause diabetic kidney problems. (Sugar is far more damaging to the kidneys than protein.) Experiments with diabetic rats show that when their blood sugars are maintained at 100 mg/dl, they lead full lives and never develop kidney damage, no matter how much protein they consume. However, if you already have kidney damage, you should work with your doctor whenever you change your diet so he or she can carefully monitor your condition.

Cut out the Bad Fats and Emphasize the Good

Fat has gotten an unfair rap as a bad guy. But avoiding the bad types of fat and eating the good is nearly as important in fighting excess weight and diabetes as choosing the right kinds of carbohydrates. Prime fat contributors to insulin resistance and excess weight—the real bad guys that should be avoided—are foods that contain partially hydrogenated oils, fried foods, and omega-6-rich vegetable oils such as corn oil, soybean oil, and safflower oil.

Some fats, on the other hand, should be considered essential medicine for those with insulin resistance. Diets high in omega-9 monounsaturated fats—such as olive oil, avocados, and nuts—have been found to be very helpful for people with diabetes. These fats increase levels of HDL ("good") cholesterol and inhibit the oxidation of LDL ("bad") cholesterol. And when monounsaturated fats are eaten in place of carbohydrates, insulin sensitivity is improved. A 2002 study in the *Journal of the American Medical Association* found that women who ate five servings of nuts a week were 27 percent less likely to develop diabetes than those who rarely ate them.

The other good guys to include in your diet are omega-3 fats, such as those found in omega-3-enriched eggs and in fatty fish such as salmon, halibut, and tuna. Omega-3 fats are needed by the body to produce fluid cell membranes that keep insulin receptors responsive to insulin.

Eating a diet rich in omega-3 fats not only can prevent insulin resistance but it can also reverse it. In one study, reported in *Diabetes Care* in 1997, fifty-five people diagnosed with Syndrome X ate a diet high in omega-3-rich fish. After a year, lab tests showed they had become less insulin resistant—and they had lower body weight, triglycerides, and blood pressure.

The effects of a diet relatively high in omega-3 fats and monounsaturated oils were evaluated in another study, reported in *Diabetologia* in 1996. After one year, people with diabetes who followed this diet were more sensitive to insulin and less insulin resistant; they had reductions in fasting blood sugar, blood pressure, and triglycerides; and they had increases in HDL cholesterol. Emphasizing omega-3 and monounsaturated fats in the diet, therefore, is very effective medicine for protecting yourself against both diabetes and prediabetes.

Drink to Your Health

Drinking healthy beverages that don't have blood-sugar-raising effects is also important. If you watch your diet but don't pay any attention to what you drink, you can develop high blood sugar and insulin levels that are very damaging.

The largest sources of added sugars in the American diet are nondiet soft drinks. These drinks have no nutrients and act like liquid sugar in the body. Therefore, they should be strictly avoided. The same holds true for fruit juices, which contain the sugars from pounds of fruit with none of fruit's blood-sugar-regulating fiber.

It may be tempting to switch to diet drinks sweetened with aspartame, but I urge you not to. The use of aspartame destroys nerve cells, and at least seventy different symptoms and five deaths from its use have been reported.

Also best avoided are sweet wines, dessert wines, and mixed drinks, which are all loaded with sugar, and hard liquor, which supplies calories but no nutrients. One glass of dry wine from time to time is usually okay, since it doesn't raise blood sugar much and may increase insulin sensitivity, but be mindful that too much alcohol stresses liver function and can lead to weight gain.

So, what are the healthiest beverages to drink? Zero-carb, zero-calorie drinks, starting with water, which is what our bodies need on a daily basis. Filtered or bottled water, sparkling water (plain, with a lemon or lime wedge, or with flavor essences) and sugar-free herbal teas are all excellent choices. Black tea and green tea are also good: they're a better choice than coffee to start the day because they can reduce blood sugar and blood triglyceride levels.

A Sample Diet Plan

Putting these eating guidelines together, what should a tasty, diabetes-fighting menu plan look like? Here are a few ideas.

Breakfast might consist of poached omega-3-rich eggs with mushrooms and red peppers that have been sautéed in olive oil and sprinkled with a little ground coriander, and green tea to drink. Or, when you're in a hurry, it could be leftover chicken or turkey from the night before and some celery sticks spread with almond or peanut butter.

A good lunch is a big salad with romaine lettuce, chicken strips, diced cucumber, red onion, olives, and a vinegar and olive oil dressing. Or try a turkey burger without the bun but with lettuce, tomato, and onion, a salad, steamed broccoli and cauliflower, and unsweetened iced tea.

For dinner, an excellent choice would be poached or baked fish with asparagus and green beans amandine (with slivered almonds) and some sparkling mineral water. Nuts, such as macadamia nuts or almonds, make great snacks in small amounts in between meals.

Tips for Extra Diet Protection

To summarize, having blood-balancing meals of lean meats and nonstarchy vegetables, with good sources of monounsaturated and omega-3 fats and calorie-free drinks, is great "medicine" to help you lose excess weight, reverse insulin resistance, and keep blood sugar and insulin in consistently healthy ranges. (If you're already taking blood-sugar-lowering medications, you should work with your doctor when changing your diet to reduce and perhaps eventually eliminate your medications.)

Here are a few tips for extra protection:

- **Spice up your diet.** Research shows that common herbs and spices, eaten in tiny doses regularly in food, are unique health boosters. Cinnamon is especially noteworthy: Laboratory experiments by US Department of Agriculture researchers have found that cinnamon greatly improves insulin sensitivity, thereby helping normalize blood sugar. That means that adding cinnamon to food, such as berries or apples, helps control spikes of blood sugar. Also, try experimenting with cloves and bay leaves, which improve insulin sensitivity, and coriander, which can reduce blood sugar levels.

- **Try cooking foods slowly at low temperatures and avoid overcooking food.** When you overcook a steak, the toughness that develops is the result of AGE formation. As you'll recall from the last chapter, AGEs are proinflammatory substances that are big contributors to the development of diabetic complications. In addition to the AGEs that are formed in our bodies when blood sugar levels are high, the intake of foods cooked at high temperatures also can contribute to our AGE load. Recent research out of Mount Sinai School of Medicine in New York has found that diabetic patients who eat slow-cooked, reduced-AGE meals have markedly lower concentrations of AGEs and inflammatory markers. This should translate into less damage to the body and a reduced risk of complications. Reduced-AGE diets in animal experiments have proven highly protective.

- **Find out what foods don't agree with you.** One way is to test your blood sugar levels before and after eating various foods to see which foods are most problematic for blood sugar control. Be sure to avoid foods that cause unhealthy spikes in blood sugar or increased food cravings.

- **Investigate the possibility of subtle, delayed-onset food allergies.** You should consider this if you experience erratic blood sugar swings (highs and lows), or if you haven't experienced improvement in your weight or in your diabetes condition after following the guidelines in this chapter. Numerous food-allergy experts have found that eliminating food allergens from the diet normalizes glucose tolerance in many who haven't been helped by usual carbohydrate-reducing means. Common allergens include wheat, corn, milk, and beans—foods that should be avoided anyway because they're high in carbohydrates. If you have trouble identifying the individual foods in your diet that your body may be reacting to, ask your doctor or healthcare professional about blood tests that check for immunoglobulin G (IgG) antibodies to various foods. There is also an at-home finger-prick test available through York Nutritional Laboratories that you can order and do yourself (see Resources).

Following the eating guidelines in this chapter should take you a very long way toward keeping your blood sugar at healthy levels. If you're still having trouble controlling your blood sugar after making dietary changes—or if you simply want to give yourself the best protection—you may need to make changes in other aspects of your lifestyle as well.

CHAPTER 4

RELAXATION AND ACTIVITY: THE IMPORTANCE OF A HEALTHY LIFESTYLE

Diabetes is not just a diet-related disease; it's a lifestyle-related disease. No matter how careful you may be with your diet, chronic, excessive stress and lack of physical activity can sabotage your best intentions to improve your health. Relaxation through stress reduction and moving your muscles through physical activity also play vital roles in preventing and reversing weight gain and diabetes.

The Fattening Effects of Chronic Stress

Our bodies have an impressive, intricate system of hormonal regulators that give us extra energy to respond to short-term, emergency stress situations. When the "fight or flight" stress response is activated, adrenaline and cortisol hormone levels rise, together telling the body to release glucose and fat (a concentrated fuel) into the bloodstream for extra energy. This works wonderfully well when we're running away from dangerous situations, such as a potential attacker or a ferocious animal.

Cortisol
A hormone secreted during times of stress to raise blood sugar and blood fat levels, which can promote abdominal weight gain over time.

When danger or immediate stress has passed, the adrenaline level in the bloodstream decreases. But cortisol lingers in the system, staying elevated to spark our appetite and make us ravenous, especially for carbohydrate and fat combinations (such as cookies, ice cream, candy, french fries, and pasta-and-cheese dishes). The hormone prompts us to refuel our energy supplies so that we have adequate fuel available to deal with the next stressful situation.

It's important to understand that up until fifty years ago or so, most daily stressors required physical responses—whether that meant foraging or hunting for food, working on a farm, or doing non-mechanized household chores such as washing clothes by hand. Kids often walked to school instead of being driven in cars, or played after school instead of watching television or playing video games.

Most of the stressors we face today are not physical in nature; rather, they are emotional or mental challenges—for example, being upset about a poor relationship, bad working conditions, or financial trouble. We don't usually go out and exercise away our concern for these challenges. Instead, we stew and chew on the troubles we're facing, and this is when the stress response becomes chronic.

The problem is that our bodies don't realize we're not using physical energy to respond to stress. The body pumps out stress hormones to increase energy stores and mobilize us for activity. But we don't do anything physical in response. So our bodies store the extra calories as fat, especially in the chest and abdomen. And excess weight through the abdomen is especially harmful, particularly in terms of increasing risk of diabetes, heart disease, and death.

Fat that is stored in the abdomen and pads your internal organs—specifically known as "visceral" fat or central-body fat—has more receptors for cortisol than other types of fat in the body. Elevated levels of cortisol activate the body to want to refuel and rebuild energy stores. Insulin levels also rise under chronic stress. So, together with high insulin, high cortisol promotes fat storage and inhibits fat release. The result is a vicious cycle of feeling hungry often, overeating, and developing an ever-growing waistline while continuing to feel hungry and overeat.

Just as our bodies were never meant to handle large quantities of foods that spike blood sugar levels, our bodies also were never meant to handle long-term stress. Chronic stress leads to strong carbohydrate and fat cravings, which leads to overeating, which leads to abdominal obesity, which in turn increases the risk of diabetes. These are all modern-day problems.

The Stress Solution

How do you break this vicious cycle to protect against weight gain and diabetes? Understanding the problem is always the first step. The second step is to stop the chronic stress response by making changes in your diet and lifestyle.

First, eating a blood-sugar-balancing diet (as you learned in the last chapter) will give you consistent, steady energy and better mental focus so that you're better able to deal with stress effectively. Many people are amazed at how much easier it is to cope with stressful situations when they begin eating a nutrient-dense, blood-sugar-balancing diet.

However, it's important to understand that stress can be your diet's (and health's) worst enemy. If you're eating a healthy, low-carbohydrate diet but feel like bingeing on sweets and other carbohydrates, ask yourself if there's anything that's causing you long-term distress. If there is, see if there's some way you can change the situation to make it less bothersome for you. If you can't, see if you can change your attitude toward it. Mind-body experts say that our attitudes toward stress influence how it physically affects us. If we look at stress from a more positive perspective, we lighten its power to do damage in the body. And when we combine an optimistic outlook with optimal nutrition and regular exercise, we create a formidable combination to combat its negative effects.

If you find yourself developing just-got-to-have-it cravings that you know are brought on by stress, try removing yourself from the stressful situation and doing something that gets your mind off the problem, even if it's just for a short while. What usually works best is some physical activity, such as going for a brisk walk, jogging in place, or turning on some music and dancing.

The Importance of Stress Reduction on a Regular Basis

Short breaks away from stressful situations work well in a pinch. But practicing ways to relax on a regular basis is usually much more effective. It's good to experiment with different stress-reduction techniques and find the ones that work best for you. Some people respond incredibly well to meditation and deep breathing. Some prefer yoga, tai chi, qigong, listening to soothing music, or taking bubble baths that contain aromatherapeutic essential oils such as lavender. Massage is usually quite relaxing and may be of special benefit for those with diabetes because it improves circulation. Exercise such as walking, which will be covered later in this chapter, is also a known stress-reliever.

The important thing is not how you lighten your stress load and relax, but that you do. When you improve your life by eating a good diet, practicing stress reduction, and being physically active, you'll hold chronic stress at bay, which in turn will lessen your risk of weight gain and diabetes.

One last note about relaxation and rejuvenation: Sleep, the body's best form of a regular time-out from life's stressors, is probably underrated in its ability to protect against weight gain and diabetes. Preliminary research suggests that people who sleep $7\frac{1}{2}$ to $8\frac{1}{2}$ hours a night process carbohydrates more efficiently than those who sleep less. People who deprive themselves of sleep, on the other hand, seem to be on the fast track to developing insulin resistance. Getting adequate sleep, therefore, is another common-sense strategy for keeping blood sugar in normal ranges, staving off diabetes, and maintaining health.

The Role of Physical Activity in a Balanced Lifestyle

Not surprisingly, the body functions best with a balanced, healthy lifestyle. Just as the body needs rest and relaxation for health, so, too, does it need physical activity.

Although many people can control blood sugar levels and lose weight by changing their diet and taking supplements (which will be covered in the following chapters), most people are healthier and feel better if they engage in regular physical activity.

Exercise helps the body burn calories to control or lose weight and significantly reduces stress and anxiety, thereby protecting against abdominal weight gain. Exercise also increases levels of endorphins, neurotransmitters that can elevate mood, reduce pain, and lessen carbohydrate cravings. It, therefore, has a positive effect on our psyche, improving our attitudes and feelings of well-being and helping us to avoid stress-induced eating that can lead to poor blood sugar control and abdominal weight gain. For some people, physical activity can make the difference between having damaging blood sugar levels or healthy ones, or between being on diabetes or heart disease medications or being drug-free.

How Physical Activity Protects Against Diabetes

Physical activity prevents, manages, and sometimes reverses diabetes by helping to correct the root condition behind diabetes and prediabetes, insulin resistance.

Insulin resistance is related to a person's ratio of abdominal fat to lean body mass. The higher your ratio of abdominal fat to muscle mass, the more insulin resistant you tend to be. In contrast, the higher your ratio of lean muscle mass to abdominal body fat, the more sensitive (or receptive) your body's tissues will be to insulin. Physical activity is of value because it often lowers body fat and builds muscle, thereby improving the muscle-to-fat ratio and correcting insulin resistance.

Long-term, regular physical activity also reduces insulin resistance independently of its effect upon muscle mass. It increases the ability of tissues to be responsive to the body's insulin, greatly enhancing glucose uptake into cells. Therefore, a person's own insulin production can gradually become more effective at lowering blood sugar.

Studies show that physically fit people secrete less insulin after being given carbohydrates than do people who are out of shape. In other words, stepping up physical activity helps the body process carbohydrates more efficiently. And having less insulin present in the bloodstream helps with weight control.

The benefits of exercise do not end with improvements in insulin sensitivity and glucose tolerance. Physical activity has therapeutic effects on the cardiovascular system that offer significant protection for people with diabetes or prediabetes.

As you might remember, the number-one cause of death in people with diabetes is heart disease. Regular physical activity raises levels of HDL ("good") cholesterol (which helps clear the body of harmful cholesterol), lowers blood triglycerides, and reduces high blood pressure—improving all of the components of Syndrome X. It also improves blood flow, which is noteworthy because virtually every complication of diabetes in some way involves decreased circulation. It shouldn't be surprising, therefore, that physical activity reduces the risk not just of diabetes, but heart attack and stroke as well.

A Few Cautions

If reading about the benefits of activity makes you want to get off the couch and push yourself to the limit with exercise, don't. Overdoing physical activity if you've been truly sedentary for a long time can be dangerous. To make sure you get the benefits of exercise without risks to your health, see your doctor and have a complete physical examination before starting a regular exercise program. This is especially important if you are over forty, if you have diabetes, or if you are obese. Doctors typically will perform exercise-stress tests that can identify previously undiagnosed heart disease and abnormal blood pressure responses. Doctors (or eye care professionals) will also check for diabetic complications, such as diabetic eye disease, by looking for fragile, small blood vessels in the eye.

It's important to know your health status so you can set appropriate limits on your physical activity. For example, individuals with diabetic eye disease or high blood pressure can usually exercise, but they need to be careful not to exercise too strenuously. Intense exertion, such as that done in weight lifting or vigorous aerobic exercise, could cause rupture of the small vessels of the eyes, which could lead to blindness, or it could cause blood pressure to rise too high.

If you have diabetes, be aware that your feet may be more susceptible to injury while exercising. Be sure to wear good socks and shoes that cushion your feet when you exercise. It is also important to examine your feet for cuts and injuries after every exercise session.

Also, closely monitor your blood sugar levels. Brief, stressful, intense exertion, especially after a period of being sedentary, can cause release of stress hormones that raise blood sugar levels and cause problems in some diabetic patients. On the other hand, regular, moderate physical activity typically lowers blood sugar levels, which is desirable for most people with diabetes. However, if you take blood-sugar-lowering medication, its combination with exercise could cause blood sugar levels to drop too low. So, work with your doctor or diabetes educator to monitor your condition and adjust your exercise program and medications accordingly.

Don't let the cautions about exercise scare you away from getting out and moving your muscles. According to a study by the American Diabetes Association, the more sedentary you are—for instance, the more hours you spend in front of the television—the more you risk developing diabetes.

The benefits of physical activity for preventing and reversing diabetes are many. It's just important to be sensible and start gradually.

The Benefits of Walking

Walking is usually the best exercise to begin with. It's the type of activity we all were meant to do, so it's safe for virtually everyone. It's also the most injury-free exercise of all. If you're really out of shape, you can start out with a slow pace for only ten minutes and gradually increase your stride and pace from there.

Many people don't take walking seriously as an exercise that protects health, but they should. Numerous studies have found that regular walking is beneficial for heart health, weight loss and blood sugar. For example, a study reported in *Diabetes Care* in 1999 found that women with diabetes who walked one hour per day five days a week for twelve weeks lost upper-body and abdominal fat, and had lower fasting blood sugar, hemoglobin A1c, total cholesterol, and LDL ("bad") cholesterol levels at the end of the study. The women who didn't have diabetes (but had first-degree relatives with diabetes) experienced reduced levels of hemoglobin A1c, total cholesterol, and LDL cholesterol as a result of the walking. Both groups experienced improved lung function and fitness.

Walking can be easily incorporated into daily living (and of course into vacations). Going for regular walks several times a week (or more) is desirable, but don't think it's not going to help you if you can't find the time for long walks. Taking several short walks throughout the day will give you virtually the same benefits. To keep walking interesting, try to vary the places you walk, such as through parks, nature trails, wilderness areas, shopping malls, and downtown arts districts.

Making Physical Activity a Part of Your Daily Life

Walking is certainly not the only way to get yourself moving just a little more. Any type of physical activity will do. To make exercise a regular part of your life, it's important to choose activities that are fun for you and that you'll want to keep doing. Bicycling, swimming, water exercises, and dancing are all enjoyable and relatively low-stress options.

Gardening is a form of movement that works your arms and middle body more than your legs and it has an added bonus: it's done outside in the sunshine. Spending fifteen minutes or so in the sunlight stimulates the body's production of vitamin D, a vitamin with antidiabetic properties (which you'll read about in Chapter 6).

Although many people think there has to be pain with gain in exercise, several recent studies show a different, much more encouraging picture: that is, integrating health-enhancing activities into our daily lives is as effective as regular structured exercise—and easier to keep up. In one study, researchers at the Cooper Institute for Aerobics Research in Dallas divided 235 healthy but sedentary men and women aged thirty-five to sixty into two groups. One group did a total of thirty minutes a day of moderate-intensity lifestyle activities, such as walking, climbing stairs, and around-the-house chores like vacuuming and leaf raking. The other group spent twenty to sixty minutes vigorously exercising—swimming or biking, for example—up to five days a week. After six months and then again after two years, both groups showed significant improvements in cardiorespiratory fitness, blood pressure, and body-fat percentage. No significant differences in the degree of improvement occurred between the two groups.

Another study reported in the *Journal of the American Medical Association* involved 1,467 people of various cultural backgrounds, from forty to sixty-nine years old, with glucose tolerance ranging from normal to mild to non-insulin-dependent diabetes. The study found that vigorous and nonvigorous levels of physical activity were each positively and independently associated with improved insulin sensitivity.

Therefore, *participating in non-intense physical activity a little more often in your life improves insulin sensitivity in ways similar to that of strenuous exercise.* That's great news if you don't like structured, vigorous exercise! If you increase simple activities such as walking and doing household chores, you help insulin work more efficiently so that insulin resistance, Syndrome X, prediabetes, and diabetes don't develop.

For most people, a flexible program based on lifestyle-oriented exercise is more conducive to long-term exercise adherence than a structured program. When you combine being more active in your life with adequate sleep and rest and a healthy, reduced-carbohydrate diet, you have an excellent foundation for keeping your blood sugar and insulin at consistently healthy levels.

The final piece of the puzzle for good health and protection against diabetes is to take supplements that can augment the effects of a healthy diet and lifestyle plan. The next few chapters will explore the many nutrients that are important for normal blood sugar and insulin function.

(CHAPTER 5)

Chromium and Other Helpful Minerals

A reduced-carbohydrate diet, stress reduction, and physical activity go a long way toward promoting healthy blood sugar and insulin levels. However, nutrient supplements can further enhance blood sugar and insulin function and provide other health benefits for those with prediabetes and diabetes.

Many people take supplements for extra insurance to make sure they meet their daily nutrient needs, but most don't realize that supplements of vitamins and minerals can offer benefits far beyond simply preventing nutrient deficiencies.

This chapter covers the health- and diabetes-protective effects of minerals. Chapter 6 covers the benefits of vitamins, antioxidants, and other nutrients.

Chromium

Chromium is an essential trace mineral needed in tiny amounts by the body, but it's extraordinarily important for protection against diabetes because it helps insulin work more efficiently. This benefits not just people with (type 2) diabetes, but also people with prediabetes, Syndrome X, gestational diabetes, steroid-induced diabetes, and type 1 diabetes.

To get an idea of how effec-

> **Minerals**
> *Elements that cannot be broken down into simpler substances. A trace mineral is one that the body needs in very tiny amounts.*

• 44 •

tive chromium supplementation is for people with insulin resistance, consider the results of one well-designed 1997 study. One hundred and eighty people with diabetes were given twice-daily doses of either a placebo, 100 mcg chromium (as chromium picolinate), or 500 mcg chromium (as chromium picolinate). The group that took 100 mcg twice a day had their fasting and two-hour insulin levels decrease, but they experienced no improvement in blood sugar levels. In contrast, the group taking 500 mcg twice a day experienced what can only be described as "spectacular" results—a drop in blood sugar and insulin levels to near normal after just four months! This was something that even medications could not achieve. But more importantly, the "gold standard" diagnostic measure of diabetes—blood levels of hemoglobin A1c—also dropped to normal.

A follow-up study by some of the same researchers monitored 833 people with diabetes who took 500 mcg chromium (as chromium picolinate) once daily. The researchers found a significant reduction in fasting and postmeal blood sugar levels during the ten months of the study. No negative side effects were shown from taking the supplements. In addition, more than 85 percent of the patients reported improvements in the common diabetic symptoms of excessive thirst, frequent urination, and fatigue.

Other studies using lower doses of chromium picolinate have found benefits for people with type 1 diabetes, people with steroid-induced diabetes, and women with gestational diabetes. Chromium is so effective that many people with diabetes are able to reduce the amount of insulin or blood-sugar-lowering drugs they take.

Chromium Is Helpful for Prediabetes, Too

Chromium supplements can also help in cases of

prediabetes. A study directed by William Cefalu, M.D., of Wake Forest University, monitored individuals at risk—people who were moderately obese and had a family history of diabetes. Some people received a placebo, while others took 1,000 mcg of chromium (as chromium picolinate) daily. After four months of treatment with chromium, insulin resistance was reduced by 40 percent. Chromium supplements, therefore, help reverse the underlying disease process that leads to diabetes, preventing and reversing the condition.

Since chromium helps reverse insulin resistance, it gets to the root of the problem in Syndrome X as well. Human or animal studies have found that chromium picolinate helps foster weight control by building or maintaining lean muscle mass and improving body composition. Chromium also helps overcome sugar-induced elevations in blood pressure, at least up to a point. Several studies have also shown that chromium can have beneficial effects on blood fats—including decreasing total cholesterol and LDL cholesterol, increasing beneficial HDL cholesterol, and decreasing triglycerides. One double-blind, placebo-controlled study found that dietary supplementation with chromium picolinate for two months lowered blood levels of triglycerides in those with diabetes by an average of 17.4 percent. Chromium's ability to favorably influence virtually all of the components of Syndrome X makes the mineral important in the prevention of cardiovascular disease, especially for those with diabetes and prediabetes who are at increased risk.

Basics about Chromium

Chromium is not a magic bullet. It benefits conditions such as diabetes, prediabetes, and Syndrome X because, as you learned, it helps insulin work more efficiently. Insulin that works efficiently does the rest.

The Recommended Daily Allowance Committee recommends 50–200 mcg of chromium per day. This amount seems reasonable for the average healthy person, but higher amounts are usually needed for people with diabetes or pre-diabetes.

Unfortunately, 90 percent of the American population doesn't obtain even the minimum 50 mcg of chromium from their daily diets. Research from the USDA found that men average 33 mcg of chromium per day in their diets and women average 25 mcg per day. Therefore, most of us should supplement with chromium to ensure that our daily needs are being met.

Remember, chromium is a nutrient, not a drug. In animal experiments, chromium has demonstrated a lack of toxicity at extremely high levels—levels several thousand times the estimated safe and adequate daily dietary intake (ESADDI) limit, which is 200 mcg per day. There is no evidence of toxic effects related to chromium supplementation in humans or animals. In fact, research shows that rats deprived of chromium have shorter life spans, while rats supplemented with chromium picolinate live 37 percent longer than they do in their natural habitat.

Chromium Supplementation Guidelines

When it comes to supplementing with chromium, there are two important things to remember: First, most forms of chromium either haven't shown consistent results in studies or haven't been tested extensively. Chromium picolinate is the form that has been the most rigorously tested and that has proven most effective against insulin resistance. Therefore, look on labels for chromium picolinate by name. It might be listed as "200 mcg chromium (as chromium picolinate)" or "200 mcg elemental chromium (from chromium picolinate)." Better yet, look for the Chromax trademark in the "Supplement Facts" label on many supplement packages—or buy Chromax brand chromium picolinate directly through the mail. Chromax chromium picolinate is the form that is best absorbed and that has been most researched.

The second important thing to remember is that the amount of chromium a person needs varies depending upon age, overall health, diet, stress levels, and activity levels. Those who are most lacking in the nutrient tend to need it the most. The amount of chromium considered safe and adequate for children seven years and older is 50–200 mcg. However, health conditions such as diabetes increase those needs. For the general prevention of insulin resistance in adults, 200 mcg daily should be sufficient. If you have any one of the conditions involved in Syndrome X—obesity, hypertension, or unhealthy cholesterol or triglyceride profiles—or if these conditions run in your family—400–800 mcg divided between breakfast and lunch may be more appropriate.

If you have type 2 diabetes, 1,000 mcg daily is recommended. This recommendation, though, comes with a caveat: If you are taking medication to control your blood sugar, start with 200 mcg chromium per day for a week and monitor your blood sugar levels closely. Continue to increase the amount of chromium you take by 200 mcg per week until you reach 1,000 mcg, and then have your physician adjust your medication accordingly. Supplemental chromium works so well at improving insulin function that, in many cases, less medication to control blood sugar is needed. It's always best to work with a doctor or nutrition-oriented health professional.

A New Product: Chromium + Biotin

Chromium picolinate by itself is very effective for reversing insulin resistance, but a new product that may be even more beneficial for those with diabetes is now available. It's a patented combination of chromium picolinate plus biotin called Diachrome, which you can order directly through the mail.

The product was developed after researchers tried to find nutrients that worked synergistically with chromium to improve sugar and fat metabolism. They investigated several different nutrients, including biotin, a B vitamin that had been found in other experiments to aid in managing blood sugar. They found that biotin worked best with chromium for improved effects.

Studies conducted at the University of Vermont College of Medicine and the Chicago Center for Clinical Research have found that the chromium picolinate-plus-biotin combination leads to enhanced blood sugar control and improvements in cholesterol profiles. Here's a rundown of a few recent studies:

- In muscle cell culture studies, supplementation with chromium picolinate plus biotin enhanced blood sugar uptake four times more than supplementation with biotin or chromium picolinate alone.

- In studies of obese rats with high insulin levels (Syndrome X animal models), supplementation with chromium picolinate plus biotin (and chromium picolinate alone) improved rates of glucose disposal compared to the rats who received no chromium supplementation.

- In studies of people with diabetes who drank a high-carbohydrate, meal-replacement-type drink twice daily, fasting blood sugar levels and glycated hemoglobin levels skyrocketed in the diabetic patients who did not receive any chromium supplements. However, levels did not significantly change in the diabetic patients who took chromium picolinate plus biotin. This means that chromium picolinate plus biotin significantly controlled some of the negative effects of sugar intake in those with diabetes.

Chromium picolinate plus biotin is a new nutrient combination that appears to be especially helpful for people with diabetes. More research with people who have diabetes using this combination is expected soon. For updates, visit the website www.nutrition21.com.

Magnesium

Magnesium is another mineral critical for protection against diabetes—and for protection against the number-one complication of people with diabetes, cardiovascular disease. Low dietary intakes of magnesium are associated with greater risks of cardiovascular disease, hypertension (high blood pressure), and diabetes. And more than half of all Americans do not consume the Recommended Daily Allowance (RDA) for this mineral (320 mg for women; 420 mg for men).

Low magnesium levels in the body have also been shown to increase the risk of diabetes. One study that followed about 14,000 middle-aged people for up to seven years found that men and women with the lowest levels of magnesium in their blood at the start of the study were twice as likely to eventually be diagnosed with diabetes, compared to those with the highest levels of magnesium. Since magnesium is necessary for the production and release of insulin, this result shouldn't be surprising.

Supplementing the diet with extra magnesium

helps raise magnesium levels in the body and improve insulin function. In one study of non-obese elderly subjects, magnesium supplements (400 mg elemental magnesium per day) improved insulin response and action, and glucose handling. Magnesium, therefore, is another mineral that helps promote healthy insulin function.

Magnesium as a Heart-Protective Mineral

Magnesium also is absolutely essential for the proper functioning of the heart and the entire cardiovascular system. It improves heart rate and arrhythmias. It keeps blood platelets from clumping together and forming blood clots, which in turn protects against both heart attack and stroke. Supplemental magnesium helps increase artery-clearing HDL cholesterol levels and reduce undesirable LDL cholesterol levels. And it's very helpful in the treatment of many cases of hypertension.

Magnesium helps insulin work more effectively, which in turn helps to prevent high insulin levels, a strong risk factor for high blood pressure. It also helps relax blood vessels. In addition, sufficient magnesium is needed for the cells of the body to maintain normal levels of potassium. People with high blood pressure—and insulin resistance in general—tend to have low levels of potassium and elevated levels of sodium within their cells. Magnesium activates the cellular membrane pump that pumps sodium out of, and potassium into, the cell; this most likely is another way magnesium lowers blood pressure.

Magnesium Supplementation Guidelines

Most people in North America pay too much attention to calcium supplementation and not enough to magnesium supplementation. Consider that low levels of magnesium in the cells (and high levels of calcium) have been identified in diabetes and all of the conditions involved in Syndrome X. In addition, emotional stress lowers magnesium levels within cells as a result of the release of stress hormones. In turn, inadequate magnesium levels increase secretion of stress hormones, creating a vicious cycle.

Virtually everyone who has or is prone to excessive stress, hypertension, Syndrome X, cardiovascular disease, prediabetes, or diabetes can benefit from magnesium supplementation. For most people, a good supplemental dose is 200–400 mg daily. Good forms of the mineral include magnesium chloride, magnesium citrate, magnesium aspartate, and magnesium glycinate.

Vitamin B_6 works together with magnesium in many enzyme systems, and it increases the intracellular accumulation of magnesium. So, to increase magnesium in the cells (which is where you really need it), make sure to take a little vitamin B_6 in addition to supplemental magnesium—something you normally should get if you take a multivitamin and mineral supplement.

People who have diabetes have greater needs for magnesium and some may benefit from higher supplemental doses. However, taking too much can cause diarrhea. It's best to work with a nutrition-oriented health professional if you think you may have higher-than-normal needs.

Another caveat: Too much supplemental magnesium can be dangerous if you have diabetic kidney disease or other serious kidney dysfunction. If you have one of these conditions, do not take magnesium supplements without consulting your physician.

Zinc

Zinc is yet another mineral important for proper insulin function and protection against diabetes.

Unfortunately, a number of present-day factors have caused zinc deficiencies to become quite common. These factors include modern agricultural and food-processing practices and the recent trend for Americans to avoid zinc-rich meats in favor of low-zinc processed convenience foods and vegetarian foods.

Deficiencies of zinc put people at greater risk for both diabetes and heart disease, according to a study in the *Journal of the American College of Nutrition*. Among 3,575 rural and urban adults, lead researcher Ram Singh, M.D., of the Center of Nutrition and Heart Research Laboratory in Moradabad, India, found that the prevalence of coronary artery disease, diabetes, and glucose intolerance was significantly higher among those consuming lower intakes of dietary zinc. The study also found that as zinc intakes rose among subjects, there was a significantly lower prevalence of hypertension, high triglyceride levels, low HDL (high-density lipoprotein) levels, and abdominal obesity—in other words, Syndrome X.

The results of this study make sense when you consider that zinc is needed to help the pancreas produce insulin, to allow insulin to work more effectively, and to protect insulin receptors on cells. The more that insulin is secreted, the more zinc is depleted at the cellular level. When zinc levels are low, the pancreas can't secrete adequate amounts of insulin, or the insulin that is released won't work as effectively as it should.

Zinc is also important because it's the mineral that's most critical for a healthy immune system. People with diabetes, as you may recall, are more susceptible to illness. Supplementation with zinc boosts immunity in a number of important ways. If you want to remain as resistant as possible to illness, maintaining optimal levels of zinc (in addition to avoiding sugar, which acts as an immune suppressor) is one of the most important nutritional things you can do.

Most Americans don't consume close to the Recommended Dietary Allowance for zinc (15 mg for men, 12 mg for women): survey data indicate that average zinc intakes range from 47 to 67 percent of the RDA. Zinc supplements, therefore, are a necessary addition to any nutritional regimen designed to protect against insulin resistance and diabetes. Zinc picolinate, zinc aspartate, zinc chelate, zinc citrate, and zinc monomethionine all appear to be good forms of supplemental zinc. In contrast, zinc sulfate, should be avoided because, in some people, it can be irritating to the stomach. Optimal amounts of zinc vary widely among individuals, but 15–30 mg daily is a good dose for most people.

Notes about Other Minerals

There are many other minerals that protect against diabetes or protect health in general. They include:

Manganese

Manganese, an essential trace mineral, acts as a cofactor in various enzyme systems that facilitate glucose metabolism. In animal experiments, a deficiency of manganese results in diabetes and the frequent birth of offspring that develop abnormalities in the pancreatic secretion of insulin. Manganese supplementation completely reverses these abnormalities.

People who have diabetes have only one-half of what is considered a normal manganese level, so supplementation is suggested. Only a small amount is needed: do not take more than 10 mg unless you're working with a nutritionally oriented doctor who advises it.

Vanadium

Numerous animal studies and a small but growing number of human studies have shown vanadium to have impressive effects in diabetic patients, including lowering fasting blood sugar levels as well as LDL cholesterol, triglyceride levels, and blood pressure. Vanadium works by mimicking insulin, thereby helping cells to absorb glucose more effectively. In other words, vanadium can help overcome insulin resistance.

A few human studies have found that supplemental vanadium can greatly reduce the need for insulin or blood-sugar-lowering drugs. Therefore, if you take any of these medications, be sure to carefully monitor your blood sugar levels and work with a doctor to adjust your dosages. A therapeutic dose of vanadium sulfate, the most common type of vanadium supplement, seems to be 50–150 mg per day.

Selenium

Selenium does not directly affect glucose or insulin function, but it strengthens the network of antioxidants that protect the body from the ravages of free radicals. This is important because people who have diabetes and Syndrome X have higher-than-normal levels of free radicals. (You'll read more about this in Chapter 6.) Animal experiments have shown that supplemental selenium helps reduce the free-radical stress that is part and parcel of diabetes.

Selenium also helps boost immunity and protects against the development of cancer and heart disease. Supplemental selenium (100–200 mcg in the form of sodium selenite or selenomethionine), in conjunction with vitamin E, appears to be good assurance against free-radical buildup and the development of degenerative diseases. This applies to everyone, but especially to those with insulin resistance.

Potassium

Potassium maintains the proper function of our cell walls and supports the activities of magnesium, a major heart-protective nutrient. If the blood level of one is low, the other is likely to be low, too.

When potassium is low, there is a greater risk of life-threatening arrhythmias, heart failure, and stroke. Eating a diet high in unrefined, fresh foods usually ensures an adequate intake of potassium. But illness and common antihypertension drugs, such as diuretics, ACE inhibitors, and beta-blockers, can promote major losses of this nutrient. If you have a severe deficiency, you'll need to work with a doctor to identify why you have the deficiency and to get prescription-strength dosages of potassium to correct the problem. Getting 99 or 100 mg in a multivitamin and mineral supplement is a good way for most people to supplement with potassium.

Some Cautions about Copper and Iron

Copper and iron are both minerals essential for health, but at high amounts they can be harmful for people with insulin resistance, Syndrome X, and diabetes. Research shows that people who have diabetes have higher copper levels and lower zinc levels than people who don't have diabetes, and people with diabetic complications such as retinopathy, hypertension, or microvascular disease have higher copper levels than people without diabetic complications. Other studies show a high prevalence of unexplained iron overload in those who have Syndrome X.

Excesses of either copper or iron can increase free-radical activity, and people with the high blood sugar levels that can occur with Syndrome X and diabetes already have high levels of free radicals in their bodies. High levels of copper or iron oxidize and damage tissues, age the body, and greatly increase the risk of degenerative diseases. LDL cholesterol, the so-called "bad" cholesterol, becomes an artery-blocking danger only when it oxidizes.

To be on the safe side, it's best to avoid supplements with iron and copper unless you have been diagnosed with a legitimate iron or copper deficiency by your doctor. However, following that recommendation, you should have your cholesterol profiles taken regularly as a way to monitor your condition. If your HDL cholesterol levels drop and your LDL cholesterol levels rise while taking zinc and no copper, you may need some supplemental copper. If that's the case, try taking zinc in a 15:1 ratio with copper (for example, 30 mg zinc and 2 mg copper). Then have your cholesterol profiles taken again.

Emphasize getting adequate amounts of copper and iron through your diet, which is far safer than supplementation. Good sources of copper includes nuts, seeds, and shellfish; good sources of iron include meats, eggs, poultry, and spinach. This should provide enough copper and iron to meet most people's needs.

A Simple Way to Supplement Your Mineral Needs

Getting adequate amounts of the minerals that are important for efficient insulin function and good health may seem overwhelming and complicated, but it doesn't have to be. Taking a good once-a-day multivitamin and mineral supplement often may be all that's needed. One multi-supplement that stands out in this regard is Alpha Betic by Abkit, Inc. It's specially formulated to help fill in the nutritional gaps that people with diabetes and prediabetes have: it contains all of the beneficial minerals mentioned in this chapter without any copper or iron. You can find this product in most drugstores and health food stores across the country.

CHAPTER 6

VITAMINS C AND E AND OTHER ANTIOXIDANTS AND NUTRIENTS

Most of us have heard about the importance of getting adequate antioxidants, substances that help protect us against disease and aging. Antioxidant supplements are beneficial for everyone, but they're especially needed by people with diabetes and prediabetes. This chapter gives a complete rundown of antioxidants and nutrients that are therapeutic for people with diabetes and prediabetes.

Basics about Free Radicals and Antioxidants

Antioxidants include vitamin C, vitamin E, selenium, alpha-lipoic acid, and carotenoids such as beta-carotene. They are so important for health that a more detailed explanation of free radicals and antioxidants is necessary to understand them better. As many of us know, exposure to pollutants—pesticides, smog, cigarette smoke, automobile exhaust, and industrial chemicals—causes the body to create free radicals as it tries to expel these harmful substances. What many people don't know is that the body also produces free radicals during many of the normal processes it performs for health, including immune-system reactions to invaders and the burning of glucose for energy. The more sugars and high-carbohydrate foods we eat, the more blood sugar levels will rise and the more free radicals our bodies will produce. Even slight elevations in blood sugar are enough to produce excess free radicals. This is a situation that's biologically similar to being exposed to excess cigarette smoke, air pollution, or radiation.

Chemically speaking, free radicals are molecules that have one unpaired electron. As a consequence, they're highly unstable. In an effort to become more stable, free radicals move around inside the body, aggressively seeking compounds with which they can react to gain an electron. They can damage anything they come across—such as fats, sugars, cells, and DNA inside cells—in the process.

Antioxidants quench free radicals by donating electrons to make up for the missing ones in free radicals. This means that antioxidants scavenge free radicals before they cause harm to our cells. They're bodyguards that protect cells from damage. But levels of antioxidants drop significantly when blood sugar levels rise, both in people with diabetes and those who don't have diabetes.

Antioxidants
Substances that act like bodyguards. They limit damage from free radicals by donating electrons to them.

People with diabetes have increased "oxidative stress," meaning they have higher levels of dangerous free radicals without adequate levels of antioxidants to counteract them. This causes damage in the body. Oxidative or free-radical stress is associated with the onset of diabetes and the development of devastating complications, including eye diseases, kidney damage, and nerve damage. But this doesn't have to happen. It's easy to turn the tide in favor of fewer free radicals and more antioxidants. Simply avoid pollutants as much as possible, eat a blood-sugar-balancing diet that limits production of free radicals, and keep your intake of antioxidants high by eating lots of vegetables and fruits and supplementing with antioxidants.

Each antioxidant is very health promoting on its own, so descriptions of the benefits of each one follows. However, it's important to keep in mind that antioxidants are synergistic—that is, they help to regenerate each other and perform complementing functions—so they work best when all are supplemented together.

Vitamin C: The Well-Being Antioxidant

Vitamin C, perhaps the most well-known antioxidant, does much to protect our health. It assists in the manufacture of stress hormones, strengthens blood vessels, boosts our immune defenses to keep disease and infection at bay, and reduces our risk of cataracts and many types of cancer. It helps to normalize cholesterol profiles, increasing levels of desirable HDL cholesterol, lowering undesirable LDL cholesterol levels, and preventing free-radical oxidation of LDL cholesterol.

As the body's principal water-soluble antioxidant, vitamin C quenches the hydroxyl free radical, considered the most dangerous of all free radicals. It also reduces the formation of AGEs, which, as the acronym suggests, age cells. And it slows the conversion of glucose to sorbitol, another type of sugar that is a big contributor to diabetic complications.

In addition, supplemental vitamin C seems to edge out some of the glucose in the system, or improve its disposal. In one study, 2,000 mg, taken daily, lowered both blood sugar and hemoglobin A1c levels. Another study found the same dose of supplemental vitamin C normalized insulin's response to glucose.

The body uses vitamin C quickly after receiving it. Optimal doses vary, but 500–2,000 mg in divided doses throughout the day is a good starting dose for most people. Also consider supplementing with a flavonoid such as citrus bioflavonoids, pine bark extract, or grapeseed extract, any of which seem to enhance the benefits of vitamin C.

Vitamin E: Free-Radical Quencher and Heart Protector

Vitamin E is the body's principal fat-soluble antioxidant. It is incorporated into cell membranes and protects cells from free-radical damage. The vitamin also limits the formation of AGEs, such as hemoglobin A1c.

In addition, vitamin E can lower blood glucose levels and make insulin work more normally, both in people with insulin resistance problems and in healthy people. In a study conducted by Giuseppe Paolisso, M.D., of the University of Naples, Italy, vitamin E improved glucose tolerance and insulin action in healthy people. In another study, a regimen of 600 IU (international units) of vitamin E daily for two weeks lowered blood sugar levels and free-radical formation among people with diabetes. It's important to keep in mind that high levels of insulin deplete vitamin E levels in the body. Therefore, people with Syndrome X or diabetes have greater needs for vitamin E.

Supplemental vitamin E is also important because it protects against cardiovascular disease, the number-one cause of death in people with diabetes. In 1993, Harvard University researchers reported in *The New England Journal of Medicine* that 100 IU of vitamin E daily dramatically reduced the risk of coronary heart disease in both men and women. Another study, reported in 1996 in the British medical journal *The Lancet*, found that among people who had been diagnosed with heart disease, the group that took vitamin E (400–800 IU per day for an average of eighteen months) had a remarkable 77 percent lower incidence of nonfatal heart attacks compared to the placebo group. The researchers pronounced vitamin E more powerful in controlling heart attacks than aspirin or cholesterol-lowering drugs. Furthermore, the study found that the benefits of vitamin E were evident within only six and a half months of when people started taking it.

Studies show that natural vitamin E (identified as "d-alpha" on the label) is absorbed and retained twice as well as synthetic vitamin E (indicated by "dl-alpha"). That means that buying and taking natural vitamin E gives you much more value for your money. An ideal dose for most people seems to be 400 IU daily.

I recommend a "mixed tocopherol" vitamin E product. This type of product contains a specific amount of natural d-alpha tocopherol (such as 400 IU), plus a small amount of natural beta, gamma, and delta tocopherols. Although alpha tocopherol is considered the most biologically active form of vitamin E, the other forms also have antioxidant properties and are believed to be of some benefit.

Vitamin E is extremely safe, but some caution is required for those with diabetes or other health conditions. If you are taking insulin or blood-sugar-lowering drugs, you may have to reduce the dosage of these drugs. It is very important that you adjust vitamin E and medication dosages in cooperation with your physician.

People with high blood pressure should start with lower doses of vitamin E and gradually build up to 400 IU, while regularly monitoring their blood pressure. People with rheumatic heart disease, in which half the heart is damaged, should start taking only 50–100 IU of vitamin E under a physician's supervision. People with "leaky" blood vessels, such as in some types of diabetic retinopathy (eye disease), or people who take prescription anticoagulants (blood-thinning drugs), could develop problems with vitamin E supplements due to the nutrient's mild (and normally beneficial) anticlotting properties. While such problems are not common, caution is warranted.

Alpha-Lipoic Acid: The Universal Antioxidant and Diabetes Benefactor

Unlike vitamins C and E, alpha-lipoic acid (also called lipoic acid or thioctic acid) is a vitaminlike substance you may never have heard of. That's unfortunate because it has widespread antioxidant abilities and is considered the "universal antioxidant." It's also regularly used in Germany as a major treatment for diabetic nerve complications.

Like the team member who can play both offense and defense, alpha-lipoic acid can act as an antioxidant on its own and as a protector of other antioxidants. It helps directly or indirectly regenerate other antioxidants—those being vitamins C and E, coenzyme Q_{10}, and glutathione. In addition, alpha-lipoic acid functions as two different but related antioxidants. Its original form, alpha-lipoic acid, neutralizes certain free radicals, whereas a form it's converted to in the body, dihydrolipoic acid, quenches other free radicals. And unlike vitamins C and E, it can act in both the fatty and watery parts of the body.

Alpha-lipoic acid is therapeutic for diabetes also because it lowers blood sugar and insulin levels, reduces insulin resistance, and improves insulin sensitivity. Supplements of 600 mg, taken twice daily, can lower glucose and improve how efficiently it's burned. High doses of alpha-lipoic acid have also been found to improve insulin sensitivity—that is, insulin's effectiveness—by an average of 27 percent in overweight diabetic patients. Sushil K. Jain, Ph.D., of the Louisiana State University Medical Center, Shreveport, has demonstrated how alpha-lipoic acid raises levels of glucose-burning enzymes and doubles cells' ability to burn glucose. In addition, alpha-lipoic acid reduces levels of hemoglobin A1c.

Alpha-lipoic acid is a superior treatment for neuropathy (damage to nerve cells), one of the common complications of diabetes. Research indicates that alpha-lipoic acid protects against nerve damage in several ways. High glucose levels characteristic of diabetes are potent generators of free radicals, and as a blood sugar balancer, alpha-lipoic acid restores normal glucose levels. As an antioxidant and regenerator of antioxidants, alpha-lipoic acid also directly and indirectly reduces the free-radical damage nerve cells are subject to. Alpha-lipoic acid also increases blood circulation, so more nutrients (and antioxidants) can be delivered to nerve cells, and it improves nerve conduction—that is, the speed of transmitted nerve signals.

Although foods such as beef and spinach are good sources of alpha-lipoic acid, the "free" form that's found in supplements may be more biologically active than the protein-bound form found in food. Animal and human studies provide compelling and consistent evidence that alpha-lipoic acid supplementation is exceptionally safe for the general population in amounts of 50–100 mg per day. Doses of 300–600 mg per day may be more appropriate for some people with diabetes, prediabetes, and Syndrome X. Alpha-lipoic acid is currently approved in Germany as a drug for use in the treatment of diabetic neuropathy at a dose of 600 mg per day.

The main caution in supplementing with alpha-lipoic acid should be with diabetic patients who take insulin or hypoglycemic drugs. Alpha-lipoic acid supplementation increases the efficiency of glucose burning and may reduce drug requirements, so people with diabetes should take high doses of alpha-lipoic acid only under the guidance of a health professional who will be able to work with them in monitoring and adjusting their drug requirements.

One last note: German and Italian manufacturers have had the most experience formulating and working with pharmaceutical-grade alpha-lipoic acid, so the highest-quality alpha-lipoic acid comes from these manufacturers. Alpha-lipoic acid is available as a stand-alone supplement and in some antioxidant formulas that contain vitamins C and E and other nutrients. It's also found in some multivitamin and mineral supplements, such as Alpha Betic.

Carotenoids

Carotenoids are plant pigments in fruits and vegetables that do double duty as antioxidants. The most well-known carotenoid is beta-carotene, which can be converted in the body to vitamin A. Both beta-carotene and vitamin A play important roles in keeping the immune system strong and healthy, which is important for those with diabetes and prediabetes. Beta-carotene also increases levels of protective HDL cholesterol and prevents the oxidation of LDL cholesterol.

Other important carotenoids are lycopene, lutein, and zeaxanthin. Like beta-carotene, lycopene (the pigment that colors tomatoes and watermelons) protects LDL cholesterol from oxidizing. It also helps protect against cancer, especially prostate cancer.

Lutein and zeaxanthin (found in kale, spinach, other leafy green vegetables, and egg yolks) are the dominant carotenoids that protect our eyes. If consumed regularly from food, these two carotenoids protect against cataracts and significantly cut the risk for macular degeneration, a deterioration of central vision that's responsible for about one-third of all new cases of blindness every year.

The best way to get carotenoids through the diet is to eat a lot of vegetables and fruits. But supplements can also be useful. Natural beta-carotene (found as *D. salina* algae in supplements) is a more potent antioxidant than synthetic beta-carotene, and it can be found in many multivitamin-mineral supplements, antioxidant complexes, and balanced, mixed carotenoid supplements sold in health food stores. People who have diabetes are at higher risk for developing cataracts and macular degeneration, so they may get extra benefit from supplementation with lutein.

Vitamin D

Vitamin D is known as the "sunshine vitamin" because spending fifteen minutes or so in sunlight stimulates the body's own production of vitamin D. Vitamin D is critical for aiding calcium absorption and promoting normal bone formation, but it also plays a major role in the body's management of glucose and insulin. A 1997 Dutch study found that elderly men with the lowest levels of vitamin D had the greatest impairment in sugar and insulin metabolism. If you don't spend much time in the sun, consider taking 400 IU of vitamin D daily. This amount can often be found in multivitamin supplements.

The B Vitamins

The B vitamins are a cluster of related nutrients that perform different functions but work together in the body. They are responsible for producing energy by extracting fuel from the carbohydrates, proteins, and fats in our food. Vitamins B_1, B_2, and B_3 play crucial roles in how the body's cells produce energy. Vitamin B_6 and biotin aid blood sugar control. Vitamin B_6, folic acid, and B_{12} prevent the buildup of homocysteine, an amino acid whose elevated level in the blood corresponds to higher rates of heart attacks and strokes.

The insulin-resistance drug, metformin (Glucophage), reduces blood levels of folic acid and vitamin B_{12} and increases levels of homocysteine. Therefore, people who take metformin should be especially careful to get extra amounts of folic acid and B_{12} and ask their doctor to check their homocysteine levels regularly.

It's always best to take the whole gamut of B-complex vitamins—vitamin B_1 (thiamine), B_2 (riboflavin), B_3 (niacin or niacinamide), pantothenic acid, vitamin B_6, folic acid, vitamin B_{12}, and biotin— usually found in a multivitamin or B-complex supplement. Extra individual B vitamins can be taken for therapeutic reasons, but this is best done under the guidance of a nutritionally oriented health professional.

Essential Fatty Acids: The Good Fats

You'll remember from Chapter 3 that there are fats to emphasize in the diet and fats to avoid. The body can make most of the fats it needs, but there are two types it can't make: omega-6 linoleic acid and omega-3 alpha-linolenic acid. We need to get these essential fatty acids from our diet—or from supplements.

Although many of us get too many omega-6 fats (from vegetable oils), people who have diabetes (and other people who eat diets laden with sugar and bad fat) have trouble converting the original omega-6 fat that we get from our diets to another omega-6 fat, gamma-linolenic acid (GLA). GLA creates smooth, supple skin, improves our immune defenses, often relieves symptoms of premenstrual syndrome, and helps maintain normal nerve function. Research has shown that supplementing with a dose as small as 480 mg of GLA per day can halt nerve damage caused by advanced cases of diabetes.

Omega-3 fatty acids, such as EPA (eicosapentaenoic acid) and DHA (docosahexaenoic acid), are heart-protective fats found in coldwater fish such as salmon, trout, and tuna. Unfortunately, most of us get very low amounts of omega-3 fatty acids from our diets. As you learned in Chapter 3, increasing omega-3 intake helps prevent and reverse insulin resistance and combats common heart-disease risk factors (high blood pressure, LDL cholesterol, and triglycerides). Omega-3 fats also reduce platelet aggregation (that is, the tendency of blood clots to form), thereby lowering the risk of heart attack and stroke, even in people with diabetes who are at increased risk. Omega-3 fats are so heart healthy that eating coldwater fish just once a week reduces a person's risk of heart attack.

You may have heard warnings that high doses of fish-oil supplements may cause elevations in blood sugar. Some studies have shown this, but others have not. The heart-protective benefits of omega-3 supplements are so important for people with diabetes and Syndrome X that I believe that they promote health much more than they threaten it. Furthermore, research suggests that a 500 IU supplement of vitamin E can prevent most EPA-produced elevations in blood sugar. So, take vitamin E with fish-oil supplements (1–3 grams of fish oil daily), work with your doctor, and if you're prone to high blood sugar levels, monitor your blood sugar closely. Also, make sure to increase omega-3 intake in your diet. If you take medications or have a condition involving leaky blood vessels, don't take fish-oil supplements unless you have a doctor's supervision and guidance.

Putting a Nutrient-Supplement Program Together

Obtaining optimal amounts of nutrients is so vital for preventing and reversing diabetes (and maintaining health in general) that everyone can benefit from taking nutrient supplements. For some people, all that may be needed is a good multivitamin and mineral supplement, such as Alpha Betic. Research has shown that a multivitamin-mineral supplement reduces infection and absenteeism in people with diabetes. Others may want to build on a multi-supplement, adding other nutrients or nutrient complexes, such as Diachrome or Chromax chromium picolinate products, vitamins C and E or antioxidant complexes, B-complex vitamins, GLA, and/or omega-3 fish-oil supplements, to fit their needs. When in doubt about making up a therapeutic supplement program that's specific to your needs, consult a health professional who specializes in nutritional guidance for prediabetes and diabetes.

Also, be sure to seek out quality brands sold in health food stores, drugstores, and supermarkets. Avoid commercial brands that contain artificial colors (for example, blue, red, or yellow dyes), hidden forms of sugar (for example, maltodextrin), mineral oil, and unnecessary binders and fillers (for example, lactose, gluten, and sugar). Products that don't have these ingredients may be slightly more expensive, but you get better value in terms of quality.

CHAPTER 7

SILYMARIN, GINSENG, AND OTHER HERBAL SUPPLEMENTS

A healthy diet, nutritional supplements, physical activity, and stress management form the foundation of a good program for preventing and reversing diabetes naturally. Herbal supplements can sometimes be valuable additions to the program. But diabetes is first and foremost a nutritional disease, so nutritional therapies should always be used first.

Basics about Herbs

Herbs were man's original medicines. Research is starting to show why. In addition to supplying concentrated amounts of nutrients, herbs are also natural pharmacies: they contain druglike compounds that can influence body processes, including blood sugar and insulin function.

Generally speaking, herbal supplements are safer (and less expensive) than pharmaceutical drugs, which often have serious side effects (and can be pricey). But herbal supplements should still be used cautiously; and people who take medications, are sensitive to drugs, or have allergies probably should not use herbal supplements except under doctor supervision.

If you want to take herbal supplements, seek out products from reputable companies that voluntarily regulate themselves to control quality and meet high standards of safety. Products from responsible companies should have expiration dates, clearly state the product's ingredients, indicate potential interactions and side effects, and perhaps most importantly, state how many milligrams of the herb or the active ingredient the product contains.

For those with diabetes, there are two herbal standouts with solid scientific research behind them: silymarin (from the herb milk thistle) and ginseng.

Silymarin (Milk Thistle Extract): Another Antioxidant

Milk thistle has long been known to improve liver function, and the liver plays an important role in detoxifying harmful compounds and maintaining normal blood sugar levels. Milk thistle is rich in a group of powerful antioxidants known collectively as silymarin, whose effects account for some of the herb's therapeutic actions.

Recent research has shown that silymarin also can have a dramatic effect on blood sugar levels and insulin function. In the largest yet conducted human study of silymarin in the treatment of type 2 diabetes, Italian researchers gave silymarin supplements to a group of people with diabetes for one year. Every indicator of their diabetes improved over the long term. Those taking silymarin experienced a significant drop in their blood sugar levels (but did not experience bouts of low blood sugar); sugar in their urine decreased; the patients' fasting insulin levels declined by an average of 40 percent, indicating a significant reduction in insulin resistance; and hemoglobin A1c, a marker of diabetic control, went down, as did blood levels of a marker of free-radical activity. The beneficial effects documented in this study are impressive, but they're especially impressive when you consider that the patients who participated in the study were very sick with diabetes.

They had liver damage and diabetes and had been receiving insulin therapy for at least two years.

Supplementing with silymarin appears to be quite safe, even at high doses, such as the 600 mg per day that was used in the study cited above. People who are taking nutritional supplements and who are not in advanced stages of diabetes probably don't need such high doses; 140 mg standardized silymarin one to three times a day is more appropriate.

The dosage that is best must be individually determined. However, silymarin supplementation is most indicated for those who have poor liver function, those who have overindulged in alcohol or drugs, or those who have been exposed to a lot of air pollution or harmful chemicals. Keep in mind that the liver detoxifies all chemicals, including drugs, so boosting liver function by taking silymarin may cause medications to be less effective. (On the other hand, taking silymarin may decrease the need for medication.) So, it's important to talk with your doctor and work closely with him or her in adjusting your dosages.

Ginseng: The Adaptogen

Ginseng is known as an "adaptogen," a tonic that normalizes body function and helps the body adapt to stress. Various studies indicate that ginseng increases the ability of people to withstand many adverse physical conditions (such as heat, noise, work-load increase, exercise, and decompression), increases mental alertness and work output, improves the quality of work under stressful conditions, and can enhance athletic performance. You learned in Chapter 4 that increasing resist-

Adaptogen
A tonic that restores equilibrium in the body and helps make the body more resistant to stress.

ance to stress is vital for combating the health-hazardous and fattening effects of chronic stress. Taking ginseng, therefore, can be an adjunct to stress-reduction techniques.

There are two main types of ginseng: Siberian ginseng (*Eleutherococcus senticosus*) and Chinese ginseng (*Panax ginseng*). American ginseng (*Panax quinquefolius*) is another species of *Panax* ginseng. In various studies, all three varieties have shown positive effects on blood sugar levels.

In one study reported in *Diabetes Care* in 1995, people with diabetes who took 100 mg or 200 mg of standardized Siberian ginseng extract experienced improved mood and enhanced overall physical performance, as well as a reduction in high blood sugar levels. Those who took 200 mg per day also had a reduction in their hemoglobin A1c levels.

Three recent studies, performed by researchers at the University of Toronto, St. Michael's Hospital in Toronto, and the University of Ottawa, show that American ginseng can lower blood sugar levels in both people with diabetes and people without diabetes. In people with diabetes, 3 grams daily of whole-ground ginseng root lowered postmeal blood sugar levels by about 20 percent. However, doses as small as 1 gram lowered blood sugar response after carbohydrate consumption in both people who had diabetes and people who didn't have diabetes.

Animal experiments have also shown blood-sugar-lowering actions from Chinese ginseng in diabetic and glucose-loaded normal mice. But the herb has no effect on the blood sugar of normal mice fed a standard diet. Therefore, ginseng seems to have a balancing effect on blood sugar, just as it may have on some other body processes, such as blood pressure.

Ginseng appears to be a supportive therapy

in the treatment of diabetes and prediabetes, but further research is needed to determine its optimal dose and which ginseng is best under various conditions. For general antistress effects, 100–200 mg of Siberian ginseng extract one to three times a day is recommended. Alternatively, similar effects may be gained from 1–2 grams of the raw Chinese ginseng herb or 200 mg daily of a standardized Chinese ginseng extract containing 4 to 7 percent ginsenosides.

Those concerned about blood sugar control can try 1–3 grams of American ginseng, in capsules or as a tea, at least forty minutes prior to a meal with carbohydrates. Tests will probably eventually show evident that specific timing of ginseng supplementation is not necessary and that regular use of ginseng between meals is able to provide ongoing blood sugar control.

As always, discuss your interest in taking ginseng with your doctor. It may be best to begin taking lower doses and gradually increase them. Possible side effects to watch out for include irritability, anxiety, insomnia, a rise in blood pressure, breast pain, or menstrual changes. Chinese ginseng is considered more potent than Siberian or American ginseng and may be too stimulating for some people. Therefore, Siberian or American ginseng may be a better choice.

Garlic: The Immune Booster and Heart Protector

Garlic doesn't just make for tasty food: it is a health-enhancing herb that has a wide range of medicinal properties for people with diabetes and prediabetes. For starters, garlic is a great immune booster. It also has antimicrobial effects against many bacteria, fungi, parasites, and viruses.

Garlic is also beneficial because it helps protect against cardiovascular disease. It lowers both total and LDL cholesterol. And it reduces blood pressure. Researchers have found that garlic contains a natural ACE inhibitor that works somewhat like prescription drugs that block the body's production of an enzyme involved in hypertension. Additionally, garlic functions as a natural blood thinner. It also can sometimes lower blood sugar levels (though research hasn't consistently shown this).

Garlic, therefore, is a versatile herb for increasing our well-being and protecting ourselves against many diseases. It should be added often to our food. Those who would rather take supplements can try 2,400–3,200 mg extract of aged garlic every day.

One caution: Garlic's blood-thinning effect could amplify the blood-thinning effects of other anticoagulants, such as the drug Coumadin, aspirin, vitamin E, and the herb *Ginkgo biloba*. If you decide to increase your intake of garlic or to take garlic supplements, consider decreasing your intake of other anticoagulants. If you are taking a prescription anticoagulant or heart disease medication, always discuss the medications and herbs you take with your physician.

Tea: The Antioxidant-Rich Drink

Tea also can be helpful for people with diabetes or prediabetes. Both green tea and black tea are rich in antioxidants called polyphenols and flavonoids, and many studies have found tea (or its extracts) to reduce the risk of heart disease and cancer. Animal studies show that both teas can reduce blood sugar and triglyceride levels. This is an especially protective benefit for people with diabetes or prediabetes.

Tea, therefore, should be preferred over coffee, and green tea, which is higher in antioxidants, should be emphasized. If you're sensitive to caffeine or want to avoid caffeine in the evening, try Good Earth decaffeinated green tea, which is decaffeinated by a natural process to preserve the antioxidants. Green tea is also available in capsules and in some antioxidant-complex supplements.

Flavonoids

Flavonoids, a group of plant compounds in grape-seed, pine bark (Pycnogenol), and the herbs bilberry and *Ginkgo biloba*, are potent antioxidants that protect cells from free-radical damage. They also strengthen capillaries and protect tissues that take a beating from elevated levels of blood sugar and insulin. For these reasons, flavonoids can be good additions to a basic nutrition program for protecting against diabetic complications, such as eye disease and nerve damage (common in conditions such as erectile dysfunction).

Ginkgo is a natural blood thinner, so discuss using this product with your doctor. The other three supplements are generally safe to take in moderate doses, but it's best to work with a nutritionally oriented or alternative healthcare-minded professional who can design an individualized supplement program for you.

A Note about Other Herbs

Chinese and Ayurvedic (Indian) herbalists have long used other herbs, such as fenugreek, bitter melon, gymnema sylvestre, and holy basil, as remedies for diabetes. Research is slowly but surely confirming that these herbs do have blood-sugar-lowering properties. Some of them also show cholesterol- or triglyceride-lowering effects. The research so far is encouraging, but more research needs to be done.

Some herbal supplements contain combinations of herbs reported to be of value for blood sugar function. At this point, it's probably best not to take these herbal supplements unless you work closely with a practitioner who specializes in the use of herbal therapies for people with diabetes and prediabetes and is knowledgeable about the functions, interactions, and contraindications of herbs.

Some of these less well-known herbs may one day play a more regular role in a natural therapy plan for diabetes. As of now, though, the research on nutritional supplements and the few key herbs discussed in detail in this chapter is much more convincing.

CONCLUSION

Diabetes is one of the fastest-growing deadly diseases not just in the United States, but in the world. The alarming rise in its incidence goes hand in hand with an unprecedented rise in the incidence of obesity—and millions of people already have some degree of prediabetes.

The disease process that leads to diabetes takes years or decades to develop. It is brought on almost entirely by poor diet and lifestyle habits.

Fortunately, diabetes is preventable and reversible. The genes we're dealt don't matter nearly as much as how we treat them. Poor diet and lifestyle habits got us into the problem we now face with obesity, prediabetes, and diabetes. Therefore, healthy diet and lifestyle habits can get us out.

A complete natural program for preventing and reversing diabetes includes a low-carbohydrate diet rich in vegetables, protein, and healthy fats; thoughtful use of nutritional (and sometimes herbal) supplements; stress reduction; and increased physical activity. Such a program helps keep tight control of blood sugar levels, which is the key to good health and long lives for all of us.

SELECTED REFERENCES

Anderson, RA, N Chen, NA Bryden, et al. Elevated intakes of supplemental chromium improve glucose and insulin variables in individuals with type 2 diabetes. *Diabetes*, 1997; 46:1786–1791.

Barringer, TA, JK Kirk, AC Santaniello, et al. Effect of a multivitamin and mineral supplement on infection and quality of life. *Annals of Internal Medicine*, 2003; 138: 365–371.

Cefalu, WT, AD Bell-Farrow, J Stegner, et al. Effect of chromium picolinate on insulin sensitivity in vivo. *The Journal of Trace Elements in Experimental Medicine*, 1999; 12:71–83.

Cheng, N, X Zhu, H Shi, et al. Follow-up survey of people in China with type 2 diabetes mellitus consuming supplemental chromium. *The Journal of Trace Elements in Experimental Medicine*, 1999; 12:55–60.

Convit, A, OT Wolf, C Tarshish, et al. Reduced glucose tolerance is associated with poor memory performance and hippocampal atrophy among normal elderly. *Proceedings of the National Academy of Sciences*, 2003; 100:2019–2022.

Dunn, AL, BH Marcus, JB Kampert, et al. Comparison of lifestyle and structured interventions to increase physical activity and cardiorespiratory fitness. *Journal of the American Medical Association*, 1999; 281:327–334.

Eriksson, J, and A Kohvakka. Magnesium and ascorbic acid supplementation in diabetes mellitus. *Annals of Nutrition and Metabolism*, 1995; 39:217–223.

Fanaian, M, J Szilasi, L Storlien, et al. The effect of modified fat diet on insulin resistance and metabolic parameters in type II diabetes. *Diabetologia*, 1996; 39:A7.

Garg, A. High-monounsaturated-fat diets for patients with diabetes mellitus: a meta-analysis. *American Journal of Clinical Nutrition*, 1998; 67(suppl.):577S–582S.

Jain, SK, and G Lim. Lipoic acid (LA) decreases protein glycation and increases (Na++K+)- and Ca++-ATPases activities in high glucose (G)-treated red blood cells (RBC). *Free Radical Biology and Medicine*, 1998; 25:S94, Abstract #268.

Jiang, R, JE Manson, MJ Stampfer. Nut and peanut butter consumption and risk of type 2 diabetes in women. *Journal of the American Medical Association*, 2002; 288: 2554–2560.

Konrad, T, P Vivina, K Kusterer, et al. A-lipoic acid treatment decreases serum lactate and pyruvate concentrations and improves glucose effectiveness in lean and obese patients with type 2 diabetes. *Diabetes Care*, 1999; 22:280–287.

Ludwig, DS, JA Majzoub, A Al-Zahrani, et al. High glycemic index foods, overeating, and obesity. *Pediatrics*, 1999; 103:E26.

Mayer-Davis, EJ, R D'Agostino, AJ Karter, et al. Intensity and amount of physical activity in relation to insulin sensitivity. *Journal of the American Medical Association*, 1998; 279:669–674.

Mokdad, AH, ES Ford, BA Bowman, et al. Diabetes trends in the U.S.: 1990–1998. *Diabetes Care*, 2000; 23: 1278–1283.

Mokdad, AH, ES Ford, BA Bowman, et al. Prevalence of obesity, diabetes, and obesity-related health risk factors, 2001. *Journal of American Medical Association*, 2003; 289:76–79.

Nagamatsu, M, KK Nickander, et al. Lipoic acid improves nerve blood flow, reduces oxidative stress, and improves distal nerve conduction in experimental diabetic neuropathy. *Diabetes Care*, 1995; 18:1160–67.

Paolisso, G, S Sgambato, A Gambardella, et al. Daily magnesium supplements improve glucose handling in elderly subjects. *American Journal of Clinical Nutrition*, 1992; 55:1161–1167.

Roberts, SB. High-glycemic foods, hunger and obesity: is there a connection? *Nutrition Reviews*, 2000; 58: 163–169.

Singh, RB, AN Mohammed, et al. Current zinc intake and risk of diabetes and coronary artery disease and factors associated with insulin resistance in rural and urban populations of north India. *Journal of the American College of Nutrition*, 1998; 17:564–570.

Sotaniemi, EA, E Haapakoski, A Rautio. Ginseng therapy in non-insulin-dependent diabetic patients. *Diabetes Care*, 1995; 18:1373–1375.

Torjesen, PA, KI Birkeland, SA Anderssen, et al. Lifestyle changes may reverse development of the insulin resistance syndrome. *Diabetes Care*, 1997; 30:26–31.

Velussi, M, AM Cernigoi, AD Monte, et al. Long-term (12 months) treatment with an anti-oxidant drug (silymarin) is effective on hyperinsulinemia, exogenous insulin need and malondialdehyde levels in cirrhotic diabetic patients. *Journal of Hepatology*, 1997; 26:871–879.

Verma, S, MC Cam, and JH McNeill. Nutritional factors that can favorably influence the glucose/insulin system: vanadium. *Journal of the American College of Nutrition*, 1998; 1:11–18.

Vlassara, H, W Cai, J Crandall, et al. Inflammatory mediators are induced by dietary glycotoxins, a major risk factor for diabetic angiopathy. *Proceedings of the National Academy of Sciences*, 2002; 26:15596–15601.

Vuksan, V, et al. American ginseng (*Panax quinquefolius L.*) reduces postprandial glycemia in nondiabetic subjects and subjects with type 2 diabetes mellitus. *Archives of Internal Medicine*, 2000; 160:1009–1013.

Walker, KZ, LS Piers, RS Putt, et al. Effects of regular walking on cardiovascular risk factors and body composition in normoglycemic women and women with type 2 diabetes. *Diabetes Care*, 1999; 4:555–561.

Williams, DE, et al. Frequent salad vegetable consumption is associated with a reduction in the risk of diabetes mellitus. *Journal of Clinical Epidemiology*, 1999; 52: 329–335.

Zeyuan, D, T Bingyin, L Xiaolin. Effect of green tea and black tea on the blood glucose, the blood triglyceride, and antioxidation in aged rats. *Journal of Agricultural and Food Chemistry*, 1998; 46:3875–3878.

Ziegler, D, and FA Gries. A-lipoic acid in the treatment of diabetic peripheral and cardiac autonomic neuropathy. *Diabetes*, 1997; 46 (suppl. 2): 62–66.

Ziegler, D, H Schatz, F Conrad, et al. Effects of treatment with the antioxidant a-lipoic acid on cardiac autonomic neuropathy in NIDDM patients. *Diabetes Care*, 1997; 20:369–373.

RESOURCES

Challem, Jack, Burton Berkson, and Melissa Diane Smith. *Syndrome X: The Complete Nutritional Program to Prevent and Reverse Insulin Resistance.* New York, NY: John Wiley & Sons, 2000.

The definitive consumer guide on Syndrome X—the combination of insulin resistance with abdominal obesity, unhealthy cholesterol levels, high triglycerides, and high blood pressure—which sets the stage for diabetes, heart disease and other degenerative diseases. Syndrome X includes therapeutic diets, recipes, and supplement plans for this common condition.

Challem, Jack, and Liz Brown. *User's Guide to Vitamins and Minerals.* North Bergen, NJ: Basic Health Publications, Inc., 2002.

A reader-friendly guide that covers the basics of all vitamins and minerals that are essential for health, from A to zinc.

Challem, Jack, and Melissa Diane Smith. *User's Guide to Vitamin E.* North Bergen, NJ: Basic Health Publications, Inc., 2002.

A reader-friendly guide that covers the basics of heart-protective vitamin E.

Smith, Melissa Diane. *Going Against the Grain: How Reducing and Avoiding Grains Can Revitalize Your Health.* Chicago, IL: McGraw-Hill/Contemporary Books, 2002.

A book that explains all the health problems that can result from eating too many grains and sugars, including type 2 diabetes, excess weight, and Syndrome X, as well as gluten sensitivity, grain allergies, and autoimmune disorders such as type 1 diabetes. Three therapeutic diets are outlined, along with information on supplements that are helpful for various conditions.

Smith, Melissa Diane. *User's Guide to Chromium.* North Bergen, NJ: Basic Health Publications, Inc., 2002.

A reader-friendly guide that covers chromium's benefits for blood-sugar- and insulin-related health conditions including diabetes, Syndrome X, and excess weight.

GreatLife Magazine
Consumer magazine with articles on vitamins, minerals, herbs, and foods.
Available for free at many health and natural food stores.

Let's Live Magazine
Consumer magazine with emphasis on the health benefits of vitamins, minerals, and herbs.
Customer service:
1-800-676-4333
P.O. Box 74908
Los Angeles, CA 90004
Subscriptions: 12 issues per year, $19.95 in the U.S.; $31.95 outside the U.S.

Physical Magazine
Magazine oriented to body builders and other serious athletes.
Customer service:
1-800-676-4333
P.O. Box 74908
Los Angeles, CA 90004
Subscriptions: 12 issues per year, $19.95 in the U.S.; $31.95 outside the U.S.

The Nutrition Reporter™ newsletter
Monthly newsletter that summarizes recent medical research on vitamins, minerals, and herbs.
Customer service:
P.O. Box 30246
Tucson, AZ 85751-0246
e-mail: jack@thenutritionreporter.com
www.nutritionreporter.com

Subscriptions: $26 per year (12 issues) in the U.S.; $32 U.S. or $48 CNC for Canada; $38 for other countries.

Abkit, Inc.

1-800-226-6227, Extension 119

www.abkit.com • www.alphabetic.com

Makers of Alpha Betic, a once-a-day multi-supplement specifically formulated for those with diabetes or pre-diabetes.

American Diabetes Association

1-800-342-2383

www.diabetes.org

A not-for-profit educational organization that provides facts and figures and basic information about diabetes.

American Association of Diabetes Educators

1-800-338-3633

www.aadenet.org

A multidisciplinary organization representing over 10,000 healthcare professionals who provide diabetes education and care.

Diabetes In Control

www.DiabetesInControl.com

A source for the latest news and clinical insights on the care and treatment of diabetes. DiabetesInControl.com is a website with a weekly e-newsletter that goes out to more than 40,000 medical professionals who educate and care for more than 5 million people with diabetes. Readers of this book may go to the website and register to receive the e-newsletter free of charge, to stay up to date on current diabetes information.

Melissa Diane Smith's Website

www.melissadianesmith.com

The place to e-mail Melissa Diane Smith, contact her for long-distance nutrition consultations over the telephone, order her books, or read magazine articles by her.

Nutrition 21

www.nutrition21.com
Makers of Chromax chromium picolinate and Diachrome, the patented combination of Chromax and biotin.

For more information or to order these products:

Chromax:

1-866-Chromax (866-247-6629)
www.chromax.com

Diachrome:

1-866-Diachrome (866-342-2476)
www.diachrome.com

Syndrome X Website

www.syndrome-x.com
A source for information on Syndrome X: The Complete Nutritional Program to Prevent and Reverse Insulin Resistance, as well as articles about foods and supplements.

York Nutritional Laboratories

1-888-751-3388
www.yorkallergyusa.com
York Nutritional Laboratories is the creator of an innovative, at-home, IgG ELISA food-allergy test, which allows consumers to prick a finger for a drop of blood, then send it in to be tested for reactions to a wide range of common foods.

INDEX

Printed in the USA
CPSIA information can be obtained
at www.ICGtesting.com
JSHW051956150824
68134JS00050B/66